HOW TO PRACTICE

SUGGESTION AND AUTOSUGGESTION

Émile Coué de la Châtaigneraie

Émile Coué de la Châtaigneraie was born on 26th February 1857, in Brittany, France. He was a **French psychologist** and **pharmacist** who introduced a popular method of psychotherapy and self-improvement known as 'optimistic autosuggestion.'

Coué's family, from the **Brittany** region of France and with origins in **French nobility**, had only modest means. A brilliant pupil in school, he initially studied to become a chemist. However, he eventually abandoned these studies as his father, who was a railroad worker, was in a precarious financial state. Coué then decided to become a pharmacist and graduated with a degree in pharmacology in 1876. Working as an **apothecary** at Troyes from 1882 to 1910, Coué quickly discovered what later came to be known as the **placebo effect**. He became known for reassuring his clients by praising each remedy's efficiency and leaving a small positive notice with each given medication.

In 1901 he began to study under **Ambroise-Auguste Liébeault** and **Hippolyte Bernheim**, two leading exponents of hypnosis. He greatly enjoyed these studies, taking much inspiration and in 1913, Coué and his wife founded *The Lorraine Society of Applied Psychology*. His book *Self-Mastery Through Conscious Autosuggestion* was published in England (1920) and in the United States (1922). Although Coué's teachings were, during his lifetime, more popular in Europe than in the United States, many Americans who adopted his ideas and methods, such as **Norman Vincent Peale**, **Robert H. Schuller**, and **W. Clement Stone**, became famous in their own right by spreading his words.

The application of his **mantra**-like conscious autosuggestion, 'Every day, in every way, I'm getting better and better' (*Tous les jours à tous points de vue je vais de mieux en mieux*) is called Couéism or the Coué method. Coué noticed that in certain cases he could improve the efficacy of a given medicine by praising its effectiveness to the patient. He realised that those patients to whom he praised the medicine had a noticeable improvement when compared to patients to whom he said nothing. This began Coué's exploration of the use of **hypnosis** and the power of the **imagination**. Coué thus developed a method which relied on the principle that *any idea exclusively occupying the mind turns into reality*, although only to the extent that the idea is within the realm of possibility. For instance, a person without hands will not be able to make them grow back. However, if a person firmly believes that his or her asthma is disappearing, then this may actually happen, as far as the body is actually able physically to overcome or control the illness.

Thanks to his method, which Coué once called his 'trick' patients of all sorts would come to visit him. The list of ailments included kidney problems, diabetes, memory loss, stammering, weakness, atrophy and all sorts of physical and mental illnesses. According to one of his journal entries (1916), he apparently cured a patient of a uterus prolapse as well as migraines. Cyrus Harry Brooks (1890–1951), author of various books on Coué, claimed the success rate of his method was around 93%.

Despite these apparent successes, many remained sceptical however. After Coué made a trip to Boston, the *Boston Herald* waited six months and then revisited the patients he 'cured' and found most initially felt better but soon returned to whatever ailments they previously had. Few of the patients would criticise him however, stating he seemed incredibly sincere in what he tried to do.

Nonetheless, the Herald reporter concluded that any benefit from Coué's method seemed to be temporary and might be explained by being caught up in the moment during one of Coué's events.

Despite these criticisms, Coué was indeed very sincere, and treated as many patients as he could, in groups, free of charge. His *Lorraine Society of Applied Psychology* was considered to represent a second *Nancy School* (an establishment centred on hypnosis and psychotheraby, set up in 1866 by Coué's former teacher, Ambroise-Auguste Liébeault). After a lifetime of work in psychology and pharmacy, Coué died on 2nd July 1926, aged sixty-nine.

HOW TO PRACTICE
SUGGESTION
AND
AUTOSUGGESTION

BY

EMILE COUÉ

Preface by
CHARLES BAUDOUIN

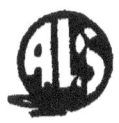

*"Day by day, in every way
I am getting better and better."*

Emile Coué

*"Our actions spring not from our Will,
but from our Imagination."*

EMILE COUÉ

TO

THE AMERICAN PEOPLE
WHO HAVE BEEN SO QUICK TO
SEE THE BENEFITS OF MY THEORIES

AND

FOR THEIR GENEROUS
WELCOME IN ALL
THE CITIES VISITED BY ME.

PREFACE

THICK-SET; somewhat short. Quiet, compact strength. A remarkably high forehead; hair brushed back, a little thinned out and perfectly white for a number of years already, as also the short pointed beard. And set off by this white when the man is laughing, almost sly when he frame, a sturdy and youthful face, ruddy-cheeked, smiles. The eyes with their straight look reflect full of the love of life—a face that is almost jovial firm kindliness—small, searching eyes which gaze fixedly, penetratingly, and suddenly become smaller still in a mischievous pucker, or almost close up under concentration when the forehead tightens, and seems loftier still. His speech is simple, lively, encouraging; he indulges in familiar parable and anecdote. His whole appearance is as far removed as possible from affectation; you feel that he is ready at any moment to remove his coat and give a helping hand. Such is the impression made on those who have seen Mr. Emile Coué, and Heaven knows they are legion, for no

man under the sun is more approachable . . .
and approached.

He is the type of what is known in England
and especially in America as the self-made man.
He never denies his lowly origin, and you feel
that he loves the masses with a sympathy that
may be called organic. Born at Troyes in 1857,
on the 26th of February—he has the same birth
date as Victor Hugo—he grew up in no more
than modest surroundings, his father being a
railroad employee. But the young man was
gifted and he was able to pursue his studies, at
Nogent-sur-Seine, until he took his B.A. degree.
Then, having a leaning for science, he began to
prepare unaided for his degree of Bachelor of
Science—in itself a fine proof of perseverance.
His first failure did not discourage him; he tried
again, and won out. We next find him at Mont-
médy, where his father had been sent by the
railroad. It is easy to imagine the boy's child-
hood, tossed about from small town to small
town of the same country, in the environment
that is characteristic of railroad employees in
Eastern France, among modest and kindly people,
obliging, humble, without ambition, laborious,
conscientious, of sterling honesty—in a word,

good likable folk. And now that the master has earned a reputation that borders on fame, it is a fine thing to find unaltered in him those same traits, the solid and sober virtues of the lower middle class. "Mr. Coué is first and foremost the type of the worthy fellow" were Mr. Fulliquet's words the other night when he was welcoming him at the "Vers l'Unité" Club. And when later he described his work as "admirable," Mr. Coué could not understand, he could not for the life of him understand—and no sincerer modesty can be found than was his at that moment.

While still a growing boy, Mr. Coué had decided to take up chemistry, but life's necessities prevented this. He had to earn his living, his father reminded him, and we sense the struggle between a scientific vocation and material needs, a struggle that ended by a somewhat unexpected compromise : the father persuaded his son to study pharmacy, which in its way is utilitarian chemistry. But that side of chemistry could not fully satisfy the seeker. Here we come upon an instance of "transference" or "compensation" such as to delight the soul of a psycho-analyst. We can picture the young man in the laboratory of his

store at Troyes, a would-be chemist but a druggist in reality, knowing that he lacks everything
to become a real chemist—special studies, experimental material and so on—instinctively turning
to another chemistry that does not require costly
equipment, the laboratory for which we all carry
within us : the chemistry of thought and of human
action.　In Mr. Coué there is a "repressed" chemist, who has "expressed" as a psychologist.　It
is well to remember this in order to understand
one of the characteristic aspects of his psychology :
it is atomic, in the old way ; it represents mental
realities as material, solid things, in juxtaposition
or opposition or superposition in the same manner
as substance or atoms.　When he speaks of an
"idea" or of "imagination" or of "will-power,"
he speaks of them as if they were elements or
combinations or reactions.　He remains alien to
an entire psychological current of his time, to
that notion of continuity introduced by James
and Bergson.　His psychology, from a theoretical
point of view, remains voluntarily simple, and
intellectual snobs are apt to turn their noses up
at it.

But he certainly returns the compliment : he
has a severe contempt—a surgeon's contempt—

for theory. The splitting of intellectual hairs does not suit him—rather would he pull it out by handfuls! His strong plebeian nature is the nature of a man of action who does not care for pure intellectualism. That chemistry attracted him is due to the fact that it is a science that calls for actual handling. And here I am led to think of Ingres' violin: in his leisure Mr. Coué is something of a sculptor and he has modeled several heads; in him there is the need of handling matter. And it may be said that he handles psychic matter in just the same way as modeling clay: in thought he sees above all a force capable of modeling the human body. So his "Ingres' violin" did not to any extent turn him aside from his line, which is rigorously simple: *his psychology is ideoplastic,* and that is its great originality.

Now Bergson himself has said: "If mind is continuity and fluidity, it must nevertheless, every time it wishes to act upon matter model itself on matter, adopt its solidity, its crude discontinuity, and think of itself as if it were space and matter." It was natural therefore that an essentially practical psychology should be this brief psychology I have spoken of. Thus, Mr. Coué's great predecessor, Bernheim, gave of "idea" and of "suggestion" somewhat crude and controvertible definitions ("Suggestion is an idea that changes into action"). With Mr. Coué, this aspect is even more marked. But while we point out here his limitations, we must not deplore them too much. They are the very limitations that thought imposes upon itself in order to become more powerful action.

It was in 1885, when he was twenty-eight, that the small druggist of Troyes met Liébeault for the first time. And that meeting decided his entire life.

Between the two men there were remarkable affinities. Liébeault was merely a country doctor, unpretentious and without ambition, who happened to be also a genius. He was the first to show clearly the phenomenon of suggestion, and he almost performed miracles. He finally established himself at Nancy, where he was to find in Bernheim the disciple and theoretician through whom his ideas were to be made known to the world. Now, Emile Coué's history was to be somewhat similar. He has conducted himself with the same modesty; he has never sought out men but allowed men to seek him out, at first a few neighbors, until now, every week, several Englishmen cross the Channel for the sole purpose of visiting him at Nancy. With that native simplicity of honest and great men, he is always surprised at this, surprised to see that his idea is conquering Europe.

After assisting at some of Liébeault's experiments, he began to study and practice hypnotic suggestion. Instantly he perceived its possibilities, but as practiced by Liébeault he found in it a vagueness that hindered his work: "it lacked method," he would say. His positive and concrete temperament, his need of "touching" and "handling" were ill at ease confronted by a reality that was still elusive and capricious. While he was waiting for an experimental and practical method, he gave free vent to his gift for observation, which is of the highest order (it will be realized how great when it is remembered that one fine day this man discovered in himself a talent for modeling heads without any previous plastic training). He is as observant as he is practical. He found the most novel, the most pregnant part of his doctrine in simple every-day observation. And this should be a lesson to us; this should remind us that the gift, artistic in a certain sense of every-day observation, is for science a rich field that should not be underestimated; other processes must be added, but cannot take its place. Too often, far oftener than is supposed, official scientific training remains scholastic: it teaches how to reason and makes one forget how to observe. We may mention, too, what the instigators of the "new schools," from Rousseau down, have perceived, to wit, the bond between manual activity and observation. A training that develops the intellectual side of man to the exclusion of the practical side, runs the risk of jeopardizing the gift of observation, which is the very basis of intellect.

So once again perhaps we have to thank fate for its hard knocks: it is those very knocks that make it educational. We have possibly cause to rejoice, not to deplore, that Mr. Emile Coué's studies were cut short at an age when they should normally have continued—to rejoice that in those years of full vigor of the mind, he learned more through playing truant than by covering the customary university programme. At every step his science plunges into the very heart of

life, and it is a very real pleasure to follow him
into that wholesome, invigorating nature bath—
a pleasure, truth to tell, which people boasting
of too barren an intellectualism no longer appre-
ciate.

And so Mr. Coué went on observing with that
penetrating, mischievous and kindly eye of his.
Making the best of things, he found in his work
an unlimited opportunity for observation. The
capricious action of remedies, the effect of a
well-placed word with the bottle of medicine, the
cure of some obstinate disease by means of an
innocuous compound, all these things, ordinary
as they are, held meaning for this great observer;
they registered on his mind during all his youth
and within that subconscious whose praise he was
to sing later, they were preparing the elaboration
of his future thesis : autosuggestion.

Meanwhile, the ideas of the Nancy school had
spread. In America they were being exploited
and popularized with all the claptrap and noise
that accompanies bluff. In that mass of very
uninteresting literature, Mr. Coué thought there

was perhaps something to be found, and his merit lies in having been able to extract the strong, vital principle from all that trash. In one of those American pamphlets which he describes as "very indigestible," he at least found indications of experiments which he had the patience to try out, and in which he believed he saw the necessary basis for the "method" he had been seeking ever since his meeting with Liébeault. This brings us to 1901. The "method" he started to apply at that time leads the subject to hypnosis by means of a series of graduated experiments in suggestion in the waking state. Mr. Coué was then using hypnotism.

But little by little the ideas which were to be his own personal contribution crystallized. They are the result of the encounter between his methodical experiments and those simple, every-day observations he had been storing up for years. What explained the capricious and unexpected action of remedies was of course the patient's "imagination." Possibly it might be that same imagination, methodically directed in the graduated experiments, that develops the strangest suggestions and hypnosis itself. And might not the passiveness, the incapacity to resist shown by the patient subjected to suggestion or hypnosis simply be the sign that when will and imagination are in conflict, imagination has the upper hand? Now this is not merely seen in cases of systematic suggestion and hypnosis. In everyday life we constantly note the same conflict and the same failure; and this happens every time we think "I cannot refrain from" or "I cannot help it."

Here we have the germ of the two fundamental ideas of Couéism. The first is that in the last analysis all suggestion is auto-suggestion, and autosuggestion is nothing else but the well-known action of "imagination" or of the "mental," but acting in accordance with certain laws and immeasurably more powerful than was formerly believed.

The other idea is corollary to the first: Since, in suggestion, it is not the one who suggests who is acting but solely the imagination of the subject, it follows that the violent and very real conflict that all practitioners have noted in suggestion and hypnosis is *not* the conflict of two wills but the conflict within the subject himself of imagination and will. Will is overcome by imagination.

This second idea, it would seem, is the essential idea of Mr. Coué and his most fruitful one. He has studied it thoroughly, with singular acuteness, and has formulated this law, which I have called the law of converted effort, according to which will is not only powerless against suggestion but only serves to strengthen the suggestion it seeks to destroy. Such is the case of the embryo bicycle rider who sees a stone, is afraid of falling on it, makes a desperate effort to avoid it, and only succeeds in landing on it with masterly precision. The same may be said of stage fright, or giggling, which increases with every effort to check it.

Undoubtedly this law could be expressed more broadly still by saying that in the conflict between the sub-conscious and conscious will, it is always the former that carries the day: Will can only triumph over the sub-conscious by borrowing its own weapons; and that is exactly what takes place in methodical auto-suggestion.

Having recognized in the imagination of the subject the great lever, Mr. Coué was led to give up hypnotism, and then to teach the subject how to use suggestion on himself. While doing this he proved that he was on the right track, for the results of suggestion so understood exceeded the usual limits. Thus he ascertained the action of suggestion in organic cases, which was also noted in independent research by Dr. Bonjour of Lausanne (falling off of moles through suggestion).

In 1910, the system formed a compact whole, and from that date started what is now known as the "new" Nancy school. At collective sittings which constantly increased in size (even the war only showed a slight slowing down) Mr. Coué obtained surprising results, and today one refers to the "miracles of Nancy." More remarkable still, this man, whose life has been a hard and laborious one, gratuitously distributes health and joy to the thousands of human beings who flock to him as to a savior.

More and more, in this great work of charity, Mr. Coué has adapted himself to the people, the simple-minded ones of the earth whom he loves and feels akin to. It is both his glory and his limitation. He lets others adapt the expression of his ideas to the needs of the more delicate-minded. If, year by year, he has simplified that expression, if he has given it that childish and commonplace appearance that disappointed so many in the course of his recent lectures, it should be understood to what praiseworthy tendency in him this fault is due.

Mr. Coué has also been reproached with constantly repeating the same thing. Well, he does. I doubt whether he may be expected to change now; I am not even sure that it would be desirable. He has an idea, two if you like; I do not believe he has three, but then he would not know what to do with a third. The two ideas he has, he really possesses; he holds on to them and he attaches great importance to them. He knows how weighty they are. He also knows—none better—the value of that concentration, that singleness of idea, which alone allows an idea to become a suggestion, a force. He also knows the value of that monotonous and obstinate repetition that he recommends for practice in suggestion. One is reminded of old Cato: by dint of repeating each day in the tribune: "Carthage must be destroyed," he destroyed Carthage That obstinacy, too, is a limitation, but it is also a force.

It is quite true that Mr. Coué's manner cannot appeal to everybody. In Geneva, especially, where everybody is so "refined," this French easy, good-nature, carried to an extreme rather shocked them, it would seem. The very tumult of success, the sort of popular wave that follows Mr. Coué wherever he goes, frightened away the mannerly and prudent. They saw in it display, quackery almost. What a misconception, and how disheartening to those who are aware of the modesty and self-denial of this great and good man! One might as well claim that the magnet makes a noise in order to attract steel, and I am sure that if Jesus himself were to return among us, trailing through the humbler streets of the town with his retinue of poor, the "well-bred" would cover their faces and exclaim "Quackery!" But Mr. Coué quietly goes on his way, knowing that he cannot please the world and his wife.

One might wish of course for more suppleness, a greater faculty of adapting himself to his various audiences. But it is best to take him as he is: a rough diamond, a kind of natural force.

If he confines himself, by temperament and choice, to action on the masses, he knows that he can do so without harm. His disciples are there, particularly his disciples the doctors, and their action can reach where his does not. Let us mention Dr. Vachet and Dr. Prost of Paris, and

Monier-Williams, who after coming to study autosuggestion at Nancy, opened a clinic in London for the application of the method. It is in England that physicians and intellectuals have best understood the powerful originality of "Couéism" (they coined the word). In France, and elsewhere too, most people refuse to understand. First the whole thing was called absurd; now that the idea has made itself felt and can no longer be ignored, we are told: "This is all very well, but we have known about it a long time; under another name it is our old friend suggestion." These are the first two stages through which according to Mr. James every truly novel idea passes: first, it is extravagant, then it is true but commonplace. Shall we soon be ripe for the third stage, that of understanding? Generally, official science's chief reproach is that Mr. Coué is not a physician, and official science tries to ignore the nucleus of doctors who are daily increasing the numbers of the Nancy school. But it should be remembered that the ideas of that school are called upon to spread elsewhere besides medicine. To the fields of education, ethics, psychology and sociology, they offer new points of view. No one who is interested in the human mind can remain indifferent where they are concerned. A few churchmen have understood this remarkably well. Not to mention the sermon preached at St. Paul's Cathedral in London on June 10, 1921, by Canon E. W. Barnes, we have numerous instances among the Geneva clergy of a fine open-mindedness which scientific men would do well to emulate.

This attitude is not surprising. Although Mr. Coué's doctrine remains absolutely neutral in metaphysical matters, it does meet on common ground with religion in its affirmation of the power of mind over the body. As for the life of the master, there is none that more closely conforms to the true Christian idea. To give of one's self as he does is more than rare; it is exceptional, and if there were at Nancy no other "miracle" than that one, it would be enough and more than enough to make us bow our heads in respect. That miracle is the mainspring of all the rest.

CHARLES BAUDOUIN.
Geneva, March, 1922.

CONTENTS

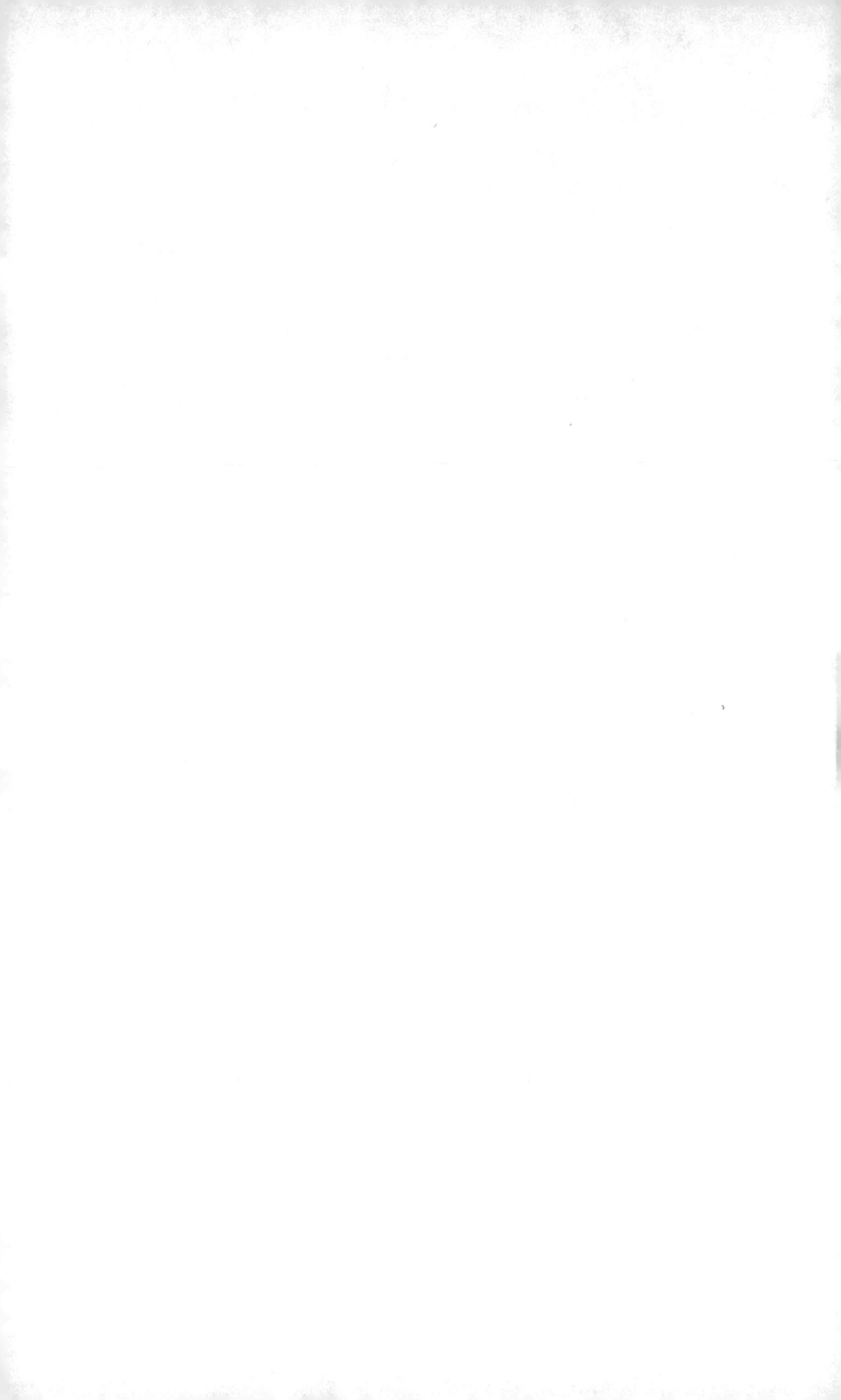

FIRST PART

INTERVIEW BETWEEN EMILE COUÉ AND EACH PERSON ATTENDING THE CLINIC AND GENERAL CONVERSATION, PERMITTING M. COUÉ TO ASCERTAIN THE STATE OF MIND OF HIS INVALIDS

All the people who are sick (they are numerous, and all maladies or nearly all are represented) are seated in a circle round M. Coué. With artless good-nature he interests himself in each one; he asks those who have tried his method to "help to cure themselves" as he calls it, he asks newcomers their state of health, gives them advice and encourages them. To those who come for the first time, he asks the reason of their visit, and from what complaint they are suffering.

M. Coué (to an honest woman who has come to him with pains in the stomach and stiffness of the limbs): "You do not walk perfectly at present, you know! Walk now in front of me, quicker, still quicker!"

(The woman runs after M. Coué round the room, and shows with pleasure that she walks—and runs much more easily than before.)

M. Coué (to an old woman who is deaf and has a swelling of the liver): "What is your trouble, Madam? You are deaf? No, no, you are not deaf because you have just replied to what I have asked you!"

"Ah! yes, but you speak loudly, that is why I can hear you."

"Yes, well there is no sort of deafness worse than that of a person who does not wish to hear!"

"Oh! but it is not that I do not wish to hear! I am deaf!"

"But you see very well that you are not deaf because you understand me! (laughter). Where do you suffer besides?"

"I am swollen on the side of my liver."

"I did not ask you where you were swollen! I ask you where you suffer pain." (M. Coué uses his method: It is going, it is going, while rubbing the painful part lightly; the woman repeats with him very rapidly the words: It is going; it is going, and feels very much better.)

A Polish man, suffering from the liver, is accompanied by his wife. M. Coué speaks to them in German.

"And you, Mlle., have you need of help?"

"You, Sir, you have a tumor on the tongue which necessitated a surgical operation. I cannot affirm that that will be cured. It is quite possible that you may be, but I do not affirm it. To certain people I say plainly: You will be cured, because I am sure of it. To others I say: It is possible that you may be cured. I say perhaps.

That does not mean that I am sure, nor does it mean the reverse."

"And you, Sir?"

"Oh! I am cured! (to those present). I was a neurasthenic for three years. I have only been to M. Coué six times, and now I am cured!"

"I congratulate you, my friend, it is a very good thing to be cured!"

"And you, Sir?" "Pain in the right side?"

"Yes, but it should go away, M. Coué!"

"And yet you say you do not use suggestion, you use it very well on the contrary!"

"You, sir, are asthmatical? A little time ago there was a gentleman here who had been asthmatical for a long time; he was able at last to go up and down stairs without becoming breathless at all. An interesting case of asthma is that of M. Mollino, of London, who had been asthmatical for 25 years, and who passed his nights sitting up in bed trying to find some means to breathe easily, which he was not able to do. He stayed here not quite three weeks, and left completely cured. On leaving here, he went to Chamonix. The day after he made an ascent of six thousand feet, and the following day one of seven thousand. He was sad, but he became happy and held himself erect like a young man. I was very pleased to see him thus. His daughter, Mme. M., also profited by her stay here."

"And you, Madam?"

"The bladder is much better. There is no longer any deposit in the urine. I am much better. But as I am a woman with a family, I wished to do some washing. I did too much, however, which gave me shooting pains in the legs, so that I could not sleep."

"That is easy to get rid of. From the moment that you felt your bladder better, you will find these pains are easy to cure."

"And you, Madam, the heart."

"Yes, Sir, I was treated in the hospital, but I left it as I entered it, without being any better."

"They told you that your heart was bad. You had palpitations? When you went upstairs you were breathless? Well, a little time ago there was a woman here, and she also suffered from palpitations. She was able to go up and down stairs without any difficulty, and you will do me the pleasure of doing the same thing presently."

"You, Madam, are very depressed? You do not appear at all depressed, you are laughing!"

"One must keep cheerful, try to console oneself!"

"To console yourself! No, you must send that away, that feeling! Do not tremble, neither your hand nor your foot need tremble, your leg too! But it no longer trembles!"

"I feel it."

"But I tell you that it does not tremble!"

"That which troubles me most, is the numbness that I feel."

"You must get rid of all that: above all no efforts."

"In the evening I am sure to be better, but in the morning on awakening, I have, I am afraid, brain trouble."

"Ah! always this fear! Good gracious!!! But you can make people die in this way. One day five or six good fellows said among themselves: "We will play a joke upon So and So. When he comes in, we will say to him: 'Why, whatever is the matter with you?' The young man in question met one of the fellows later, and the latter said to him: 'Why, whatever is the matter with you today? Are you ill? You look so strange!' He replies: 'No, I am not ill, no . . . there is nothing wrong with me.' Later he met another

of his friends who said to him: 'But you are as
yellow as a guinea! Are you ill? You look so
anyhow!' The poor fellow hesitated and said:
'No . . . I . . . I have nothing the matter with
me; but it is odd, some one else told me almost
the same thing.' When the third man speaks to
him, he believes himself ill, and when the fourth
and fifth, he really is ill and goes to bed. . . . !"

"And you, Sir, neurasthenia? Ask this gentleman the formula for healing yourself. He will
tell you all about it presently. He was completely
cured himself.

"I do not sleep!"

"You will sleep like a doormouse, and then
everything will assume a rosy tint. There is a
certain expression in your face which shows that
it will soon leave you, and if you can smile there
is no longer any neurasthenia!"

"I can no longer write; I cannot write or speak
quickly; I am sad and can no longer think. I
am losing my faculties!"

"Ah, well, you can no longer think! The best
proof that you can still think is that you say (and
in consequence you think it) 'I can no longer
think.' I am going to give you a prescription
which will make you laugh, but which is excellent.

Every time that you have gloomy thoughts, you will place yourself in front of a looking glass, and laugh at yourself. In a few minutes you will find that you are laughing quite naturally, as you are doing now. And when you can laugh as you are at present, neurasthenia goes away. I tell you NEURASTHENIA GOES AWAY."

"And you, Madam?"

"My pains are better. Every time that I have them, I use the method you have shown me, but they come back!"

"Ah! Well, you must not forget this, that I never cure anyone. For the moment you are not getting well very fast. Very good. Then say to yourself: 'After all it is not so bad today, and tomorrow it will be still better. . . .' "

"And you, Madam, the stomach? You cannot digest your food? Well, well, you will digest your food soon."

"I wish to conquer my fear."

"Ah! You are frightened of being afraid, and yet it is the fear of being frightened that makes you afraid!"

"And you, Madam. You say that during the day you feel well?"

"Yes, it is in the night I feel bad; I feel stifled and expectorate a lot."

"You are careful to make your suggestions?"

"I never miss."

"Then you will be cured."

"And you, Madam. You continue to improve. No one will recognize you when you return to London! Madame came here in a deplorable state of mind. She had to have some one with her lest she should throw herself overboard while on the boat. She imagined a whole host of things. But she started imagining just the contrary, and you see the result. And Madame, has only been here a fortnight."

"And you, Mlle., you continue to get better?"

"Oh, yes, the other day my friend left me, and I did not shed a single tear, in fact I wanted to laugh!"

"Oh, but you are exaggerating, you must be hardhearted. It is good, however. You have made progress."

"(To an English woman who has a trembling) And you, well and good, are better. It seems that yesterday you were able to get up from your chair and walk fairly well . . . not this morning? But if you are able to do it one day, you can do it

every day. You must always say to yourself:
'I can.' You cannot walk well today? Well,
presently you are going to run! It is not hope
that will cure you. It is the certainty."

(A voice in the audience.) "I saw Mlle. get
out of the tram almost without help. One held
out a hand to her, because one is used to helping
her, and so Mlle. took it but she could have done
without it."

"Ah! but you have deceived me, Mlle., that is
naughty of you!"

To a young girl who had not been able to see
at all with the left eye, and whom M. Coué has
cured.) "Come, Mlle., let us measure your sight!"
(M. Coué moves further and further from her,
until she can no longer see his features plainly.)
"But you have made great progress! Soon you
will be able to see a fly upon a cathedral!" (A
voice.) "I told Mlle. she would soon be able
to see the Cannebiere from here!" (Laughter.)

"Well, Mlle., if you had continued to use your
lorgnon, you would have become quite blind in
time. You owe me a candle at least. (To the
assembly.) "Since Mlle. was two years old
(she is now twenty-two) she could no longer
see with the left eye as a result of meningitis.

For a whole year this eye was bandaged. As she was a whole year thus and not able to see anything, the idea fixed itself in her mind: 'I cannot see!' When the bandage was removed she could not see at all with that eye. I just said that she might have become completely blind, because she was overstraining the right eye, and that if she were not careful, she would end by not seeing at all. But now Mlle. who could not play the piano for more than five minutes, can play for two hours, and she sews and reads with the left eye."

"And you, Mme., always the same thing? But you walk very well! Therefore it is not the same thing. Above all, do not get the idea into your head that you are not improving, you MUST improve. It is perfectly normal for you to do so!"

"And you, young man, your cold? You have not lost it? It is that you are too fond of it, you know! You no longer have any boils or pimples. They become fewer and fewer? So much the better."

(An English lady.) "M. Coué, will you help me to cure my left eye, and my throat which is contracted?"

"You say, Madam, that your throat is contracted. That will relax. It is a nervous affection. You say that you had an incision the result of an operation? But do you always have the same sensations? Sometimes it is stronger and at other times less? There is then something else beside the incision. If it were caused exclusively by the incision, you would always have the same feeling. It is partly a psychological affection with you. The other day there was a little man here who could hardly speak. At the end of the séance he could speak nearly normally. It must have been continued for he did not return . . . and generally when people do not come to see me again, it is because they are cured!"

(During the séance the following day.)

(M. Coué, to a person suffering with her throat.) "And you, Madam, who had contraction of the throat, were you able to make a sound yesterday?" "I sang, but it was horrible, really frightful."

"You should not have begun by singing; you should have started by trying one or two notes on the piano and singing with it. Once a person is persuaded that they can sing one note, although they did not think they were capable of doing so, they can sing other notes."

"And you, Madam! You tell me that you had a pretty voice up to the age of 14 years, and that they burnt your vocal cords following an operation? From this account, I do not say that you will recover a pretty voice, because your voice is hoarse. You must not do too much talking, and your voice may lose its hoarseness."

(A voice.) "I know a young girl who gave herself the suggestion that she should have a pretty voice. Is it possible?"

"Yes, it is possible."

(To a man who enters.) "You have come to look on? No, for help? Good! I will teach you how to use an instrument which you possess when you are no longer here! You are neurasthenic? You may not be cured all at once. When Christ carried His cross He fell more than once. And so we mortals are also allowed to fall sometimes. But you will be quite cured in time.

"For twenty years I have not slept!"

"Ah, well, when you really understand my treatment, you will sleep like a doormouse, you will see!"

"I was under Bernheim. He tried to make me sleep, but he was not able to do so."

"It is not practical to make people sleep, because if you are not successful, they say that as they cannot be cured! Therefore I send no one to sleep."

"With me it depends upon the weather, the wind. This weather is bad for me. I had a very bad day. I got up very tired and depressed. I knew at once that the weather was going to change!"

"Well, I cannot tell the weather beforehand (maliciously) that is unless I look at the sky! (Laughter.) But the time will come when you will no longer be dependent upon the wind and the weather!"

(A young girl in the assembly.) "I was afraid to be in the streets in Paris. I was afraid to go out, of the noise, and my heart used to beat. From the first time on leaving here, I was no longer frightened. Then I was given the management of a studio for drawing. I had no ideas and was without imagination. I was terrified to enter the studio! Now I have imagination and ideas. I go to my work with pleasure!"

"I have seen at M. Vachet's clinic at Paris, a man who could not go out unless he was accompanied like a child, by a person who held either his hand or his coat. When he left the doctor's, he went on foot and alone along the road from Fontaine St. Michael to the Grand Boulevards."

(To an Englishwoman.) "And you, Mlle., you have just returned from your little journey?

"Yes, M. Coué. Yesterday in the train there was a young girl who complained to me of having bad headaches; I told her they could be cured, and explained to her what you have told me. She listened very carefully, and after a treatment her headache vanished. When she left she had no pain at all."

"I am very pleased to hear that!"

(A voice.) "But there are some people who are cured at once, while others take a much longer time!"

"Because it is too easy to understand! There are those who cannot imagine so simple a thing will produce such an effect!"

(The Englishwoman continues.) "After that, we went to a cottage, and the woman there suffered from varicose veins; we did the same thing to her and she found relief. She was paralyzed on one side, and had an irritible rash on the left side of her face. She did not tell us about her left eye which was very weak. We used the same method, and when we had finished, not only did

she feel much better, but upon opening her eyes
she said: 'But I can see quite well with that eye!'
We did not know when we started to treat her
that her eye was bad, but her unconscious Self
had done what was necessary to improve her
sight!"

(To a child suffering from nervous attacks.)
"And you, my little friend, have you made your
suggestion well? You tell me, Mme., that he only
has attacks every two or three months? You
consider them getting better? Good! But it is
necessary that either you or your husband continue to make suggestions to him at night. I am
quite sure that he will be completely cured in
time."

"And you, Mme., have you made your obses-
sions of yesterday pass? Very good! Autosuggestion is just a trick! As soon as you begin to
suffer either physically or mentally do not let it
get worse. You must never let anything get the
better of you. That is what Horace meant when
he said: 'Let nothing overcome you'!"

"And you, Madam?"

"I was much better, but the doctor told me it
was my nerves. He said to me: 'Go and see M.
Coué; it is only he who can cure you!'"

"He said I could cure you? It is not I who cure you. I show you the method to use. I can do nothing of myself; although you may believe it of me. It is for you to use the method which I give you. If you are not cured, you must not say that it is I who failed. It is you who have failed if you are not able to cure yourself with the method I have shown you."

"And you, Madam, for this little one?"

"His leg is twisted since he had convulsions when he was a year old."

"Walk a little way; he limps a little." (The child walks but limps.)

"Yes, he has coxalgia, one leg is a little shorter than the other. Does it hurt when you walk? No? If there is no pain, his lameness is due to the fact that one leg is shorter than the other. It is thinner than the other, you say? Yes, because it does not get the same amount of nourishment. Yesterday there was a young man here who had one leg atrophied. He found that he had made progress, however, because though his leg was not yet a normal size, the calf was nearly as big as that of his other leg."

(A voice.) "One would say that this child's leg is crooked."

"His leg will get better, very probably, but it needs time. It has to build up new muscles."

"And you, Mlle., you very often have a headache? Nearly every day? You will see how quickly a headache can disappear!"

(A woman.) "I was the same when I was a girl; I had a headache every Sunday. (Smiles.) Yes, I used to say to myself all the week: 'Oh, how I am going to suffer again next Sunday! And from Sunday to Sunday I expected the pain; at 9 o'clock I expected the pain and it used to come!"

"And now?"

"Now I have no time to think about it. I am married and have too much to do!"

"And you, Sir, you have pains between the ribs and inflammation of the ear? You have completely lost the hearing on that side? Then I cannot affirm that you will be completely cured, but it is quite possible; is there still a discharge from it? Probably under the influence of autosuggestion, your unconscious Self will do what is necessary to heal the lesions, and as they heal, the hearing may return. As an example, a man who had been pensioned off by the railroad company, had both ear drums perforated, and was as deaf as a post! He was cured and could hear not so well as formerly perhaps, but sufficiently well to enable him to hear me when I spoke to him as I am doing to you at this moment."

"The liver, Mme.? Hepatic colic? When you have hepatic colic that comes because the liver is not functioning properly; it is secreting an acid bile instead of an alkaline bile. Gallstones? You have not got them now, if you had you would be as yellow as a guinea! When the bile is acid, it leaves a deposit in the bile duct, a thick cholisterine fluid, which accumulates and forms gallstones; it follows that if you have a collection of these gallstones they do not dissolve, and every time they pass into the canal leading to the gall bladder, they cause pain and colic; but once they are used up they will not form again. As to the metritis, that can be cured and should do so rapidly; the first case of metritis I saw was of 24 years standing, they wished to operate upon this person but she was cured very quickly."

"A varicose ulcer? That is not easily cured by ordinary treatment, but you can do so easily by autosuggestion."

"I always put on my ointment and bandage."

"Yes, well put on a little suggestion ointment instead. You have had it for some time?"

"It was 10 years ago, but it got well; then 8 months ago I knocked my leg badly and it opened again. I have only been to you three times, and yet I am cured! The skin is still thin, of course, but I am cured!"

"And you, Mme., you always have gloomy thoughts?"

"Yes, every time I wake up in the morning I feel like going and drowning myself!"

"Ah! well, you will soon drown yourself in joy instead of grief!"

(A woman.) "I, Sir, have already been to you this summer and I was quite cured, but I forgot to continue my suggestion, and so am obliged to come and see you."

"And if I were unkind I should tell you that it served you right! It is such a simple thing to make this little suggestion night and morning; you do not forget your meals; forget sometimes to have your dinner, but make your suggestions regularly."

(A woman suffering from eczema.) "My hands are very bad! (she shows them all cracked, etc.) I have had it since I was fourteen years old."

"One thing you must not do is to put your

hands in water with soap or soda; you must not wash your hands at all in the usual way; you must smear them well with a little pad of wadding dipped in oil, and then take your own special towel to wipe your hands upon; but if you continue to put your hands in water, you will make your suggestion in vain; it would return and you would scratch your hands with your nails!"

"And you, my friend?"

"It is nervousness, I stammer."

"You are sure that you stammer? Well, I say that you do not! Say: "Good day," you see you do not stammer! Say: I am sure to get well! You have only got to think that you will not stammer and you will no longer do so. I have seen half-a-dozen stammerers who do not stammer before me; it is only because I make them say: "I will stammer no more! One day a young man came to me and said: I have come to you because I stammer. I asked him: Is it your intention to make fun of me? You do not stammer at all! He replied: But I used to. . . . Ah! Well, I told him, as you have not stammered to-day you will never stammer any more. And for you, Sir, it is the same thing; above all do not fear to stammer and you will be all right."

"And you, Sir, rheumatism?"

"It begins in the calf and goes up to the knee; when I am in bed it does not hurt so much, but I find it very difficult to walk."

"And suppose I tell you that you will walk easily presently?"

"I wish I could, and above all be able to run with the beagles."

"You, Mme., have stage-fright? At Paris I saw a young girl who taught the piano, violin and singing; she had the same thing, but she came to me and was cured at once; she became as bald as a billiard ball with the fright she endured the day of the examinations! Very often when the examinations are going to take place the pupils from the Conservatories and elsewhere come to me; and it is very seldom that it fails. Understand clearly that it is the idea of fear which produces it; you have stage-fright because you fear to have it; when you go to address a meeting you must say to yourself: I am superior to all these people, I am going to teach them something, I am the teacher, these are the pupils!

In these conditions one does not have stage-fright."

"You, Sir, have a piece of shrapnel in the calf of the leg? It worries you when you are resting? Has it been removed? No, and it gives you cramp; that is easy to get rid of!"

"As for you, Mlle. You are very timid and nervous! You should become completely of yourself! What age are you? Seventeen years? It is necessary for you, Madame, to give her suggestions at night; when the child is asleep, approach her bed very quietly, and when about a yard distant speak very low to her so as not to awaken her, and repeat 20 or 25 times those things which you wish her to obtain, so that they may enter into her unconscious Self; for there are two individuals within us, the conscious and the unconscious Selves. When we sleep the conscious Self sleeps, but the unconscious Self is awake and it is to him we speak."

"You are better I can see!" (to a man suffering with his chest).

"Yes, and I am eating better!"

"And your expression has changed; you have the look of a human being who has taken on a new lease of life!"

(A woman.) "I turn giddy constantly; when I see a motor car I want to get out of its way, but I cannot! This is caused by the fact that one day in trying to avoid a tram, I was nearly run over by a motor bus."

"But Mme. I too, should become stuck, if on seeing a motor coming I were to say to myself: I am stuck, I cannot move! Listen; you are on a road, suddenly you hear a chuff, chuff, chuff! You turn round and perceive a car coming along at a hundred miles an hour! If you are unfortunate enough to say to yourself: I want to save myself, but I cannot! There you are! And if the chauffeur says: Good gracious! I am going to run over her . . . it happens! If on the contrary, he does not lose his head, he gives the little turn that is necessary and misses you! You must not say: I want to save myself! But: I can save myself! There is a great difference!"

(Another woman.) "I always have an inflammation of the brain caused by a cold, and I cannot get rid of it."

"Ah, Mme., you are wrong to speak in that way, you must never say that! Say that which is true, and which will become all the more quickly

and completely true the more often you think it:
I am on the way to recovery!"

"And you, Mme?"

"It is this bad time of year that brings me to
you; as soon as I am in the street, my eyes fill
with water; I have tried lotions . . . everything!"

"Ah! Well, now you will try an infusion of
suggestion and you will see! Tell yourself firmly
that your eyes will not fill with water when you
go out and they will not!"

"And you? Sciatica? Well you must leave it
behind you here! I shall be very happy to receive
it, and I will throw it into the rubbish basket!"

"I shall be only too pleased to leave it with
you!"

"And you, a sore throat? You must make
your suggestions regularly and calmly; there are
two conditions necessary for suggestions to work
well; first, you must make it with the certainty
that it will make your trouble disappear, and
secondly you must make it without effort; if you
fail it is because you have made efforts, and then
you obtain exactly the contrary of that which
you desire."

"You, the blues!"

"They tell me it will go away."

"So it will, and then you can wish it a pleasant journey!"

(A voice.) "What is it, the blues?"

"Sad and gloomy thoughts."

(A man.) "I, Sir, have pains everywhere; all I can think of is how I suffer."

"Those are very fine ideas! You must not think thus! I say this to all: as soon as you feel a pain, put it very politely outside the door, with all the ceremony due to it; think of your pain if you like, but set it at defiance by saying to it: Ah! my friend, up to the present it is you who have had a hold on me, but from now onwards it is I who have a hold upon you!"

*

* *

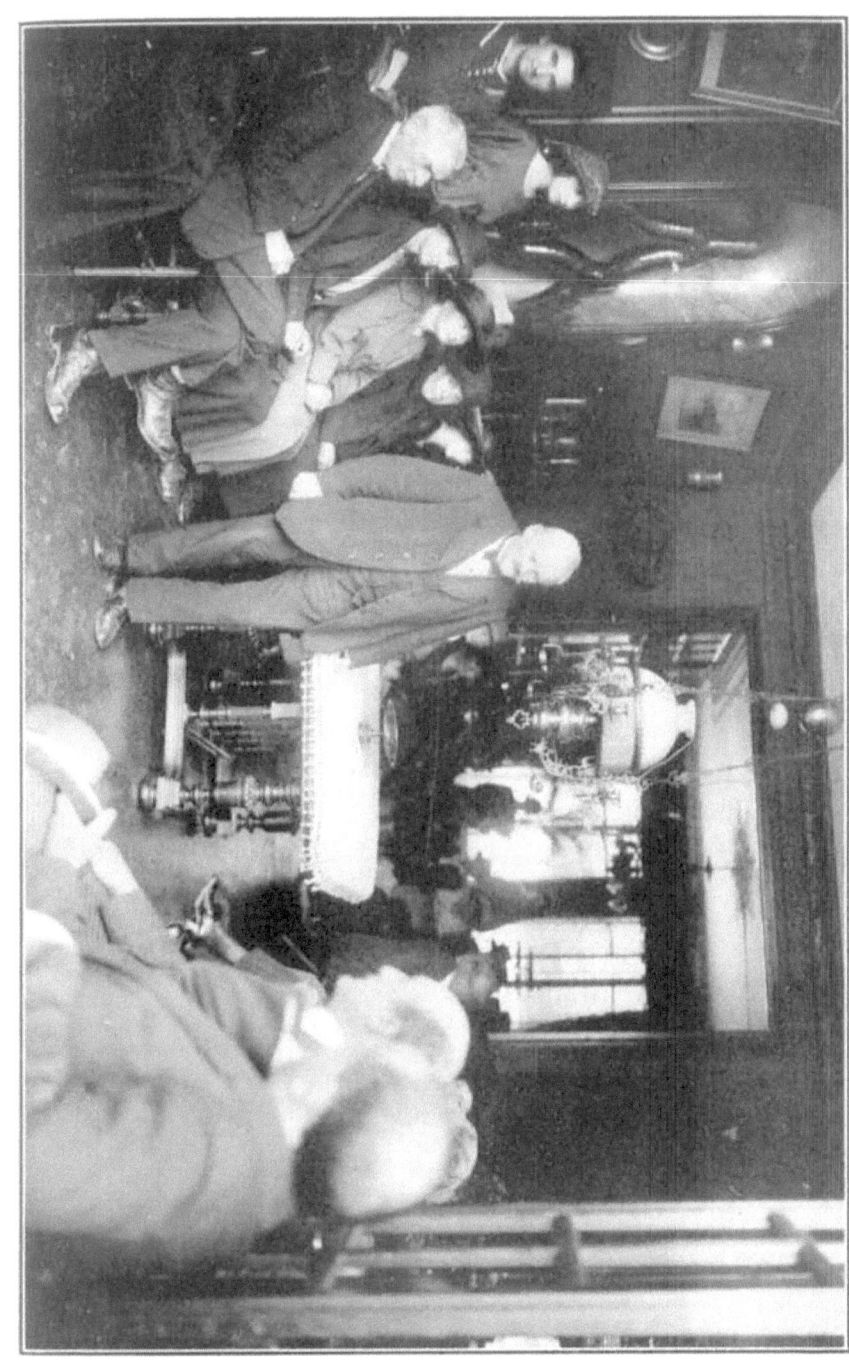
Coué Conducting a Clinic in his House

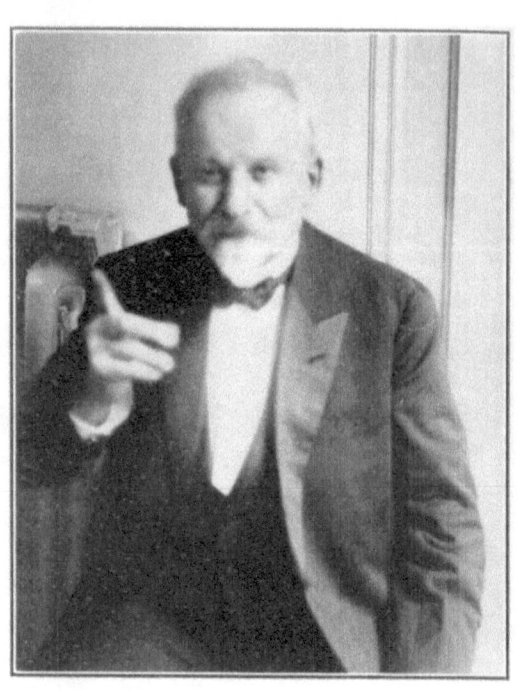

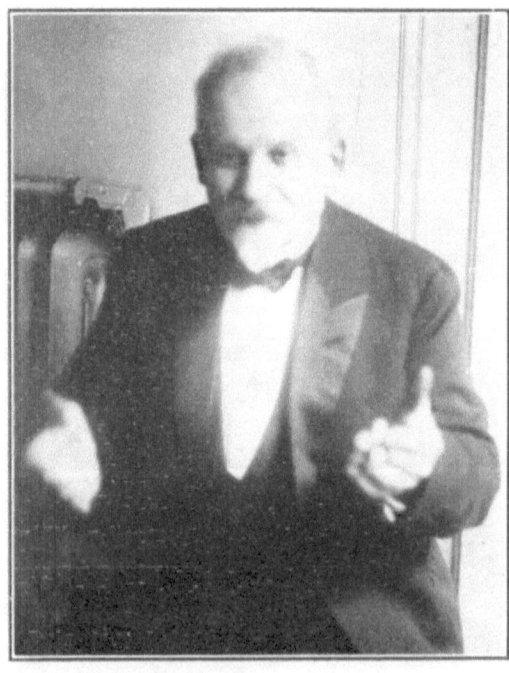

Courtesey Cleveland Plain Dealer

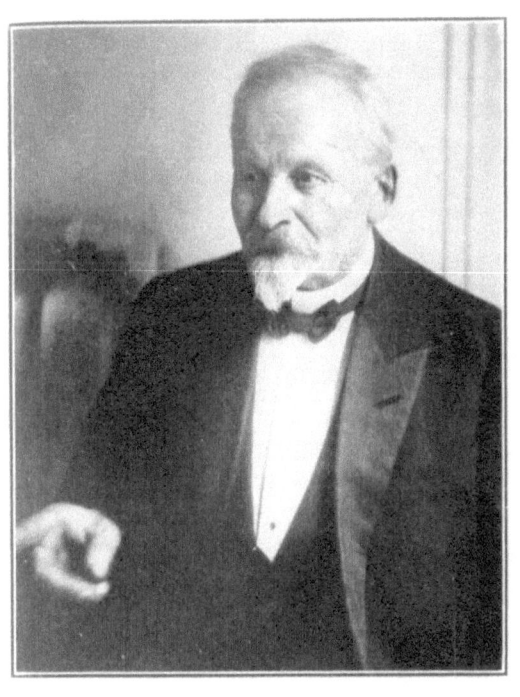

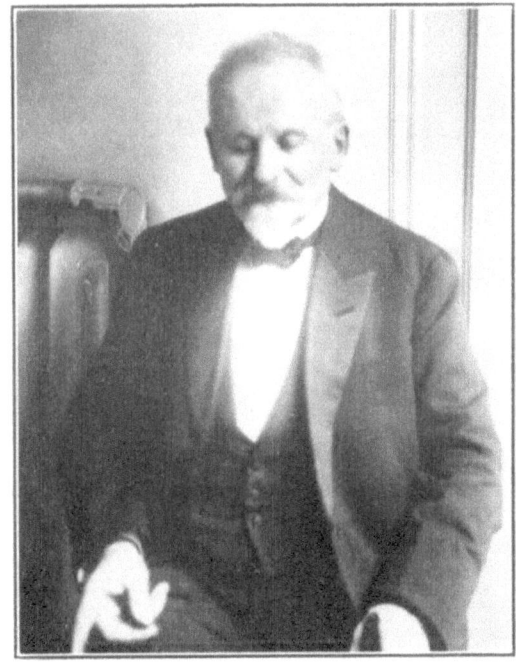

Coué and Patients in his Garden

SECOND PART

EXAMPLES A N D EXPERIMENTS
WHICH SHOW TWO THINGS:
FIRSTLY, THAT EVERY IDEA THAT
WE PUT INTO THE MIND BECOMES
A REALITY (WITHIN THE LIMIT
OF POSSIBILITY, BE IT UNDER-
STOOD). SECONDLY, THAT CON-
TRARY TO WHAT IS GENERALLY BE-
LIEVED, IT IS NOT THE WILL
WHICH IS THE FIRST FACULTY OF
MAN, BUT THE IMAGINATION.

M. Coué speaking to new patients:

"I am going to explain to you in a few words what autosuggestion is. Presently I am going to demonstrate to you two things, by certain experiments which some of you have already made, and then upon those who have not yet done so.

"The first of these two points is this: Whatever idea we put in our mind, never mind what that idea may be, becomes true for us, even if it be actually untrue. The same occurrence seen by ten different persons is seen from ten different points of view. Thus when a crime is committed, you may have thirty persons who have witnessed it. Good! From the witness box at the trial, you will hear thirty different accounts, because none of the persons have seen the act from the same aspect. To one it appears white, to another black.

"Further, every idea that we put into the mind becomes a reality in so far as it is within the realms of possibility, naturally (I make this reservation, because if we think a thing that is impossible—such as having lost a leg that a new one

59

will grow in its place—there is no chance that such an idea will be realized.) But if we put a thought in the mind that is possible, it becomes a reality for us. Thus you think: I do not sleep at night, and you do not sleep! What is insomnia? It is the idea that when you go to bed, you will not sleep! The person who sleeps well at night is the person who knows very well that in going to bed, he will sleep well! It is sufficient to think: I am constipated, to become constipated! It is the idea that we have that unless we take such and such a medicine, we shall not have an evacuation of the bowels every day. It is true, for if some-one were to introduce surreptitiously into your box of pills or cachets, cachets containing starch or bread pills, having the identical outward ap-pearance of your usual cachets or pills, your bowels would work in exactly the same manner as if you had taken your pill of extract of rhubarb, or a cachet containing cascara! But of course, only on the condition that you knew nothing whatever about it! It is the same with those injections of distilled water that they give to patients, telling them that they are injections of morphia! They believe that it is morphia and they feel relieved! It is sufficient to think: it has frozen after the thaw, I am sure to fall! If you say that, you may be quite certain of the result! Those who have no fear of falling do not fall.

"You see the importance of this point, because as every idea that we put in the mind becomes a reality (in the realm of possibility) if, being ill either physically or otherwise, we put in our minds the idea that we can be cured, we become cured!

"The second thing that these experiments will show is, that contrary to that which is generally accepted, it is not the WILL which is the first faculty of man, but the IMAGINATION. We say we can do everything by the will; I am going to show you that such is not the case; every time that there is a conflict between the will and the imagination, not only do we not do that which we wish, but we do exactly the contrary! If, being unable to sleep during the night, you make no efforts to go to sleep, you remain calm and quiet in your bed; but if you have the misfortune to try and make efforts to do so, you toss and turn from side to side, cursing and swearing! You get into an overexcited condition, instead of one of repose which you seek. Your state of mind is: I WILL go to sleep, but I CANNOT!

You obtain the contrary of that which you seek!
This is the example of insomnia.

SECOND EXAMPLE.   Forgetting a name.
You say: I will remember the name of Mrs. . . .
but I CANNOT! I have forgotten it! And
you do not remember it; then you say to
yourself: I shall remember it presently! And as
a matter of fact, the idea in your mind: I have
forgotten; is replaced by the idea: I shall remember, and you interrupt yourself later in conversation to say: Ah! It was Mrs. So and So of whom
I wished to speak!

THIRD EXAMPLE.   Uncontrollable laughter.   You must have all noticed the greater the
efforts you make not to laugh, in certain circumstances the more impossible it becomes, and
the louder you laugh! State of mind: I WILL
stop laughing, but I CANNOT!

FOURTH EXAMPLE.   A cyclist learning to
ride.   He is on the road; he perceives an obstacle
in the distance, a stone, a dog, etc., and says to
himself: Whatever happens I WILL not run into
it! He bends over the handle bars for fear of
running into the obstacle, but the greater the efforts he makes to avoid it, the more surely does

he run into it! State of mind: I WILL avoid that obstacle, but I CANNOT.

FIFTH EXAMPLE. The stammerer. The more a person who stammers tries to speak normally, the more he stammers! If he says to himself: Now I must say good-day, but I WILL not stammer! he will find that he will stammer all the more, and he starts ten times! State of mind: I WILL stop stammering, but I CANNOT!

"Therefore I repeat, that every time the WILL and the IMAGINATION come in conflict, not only can we not do that which we wish, but we do precisely the contrary. Because we have within us two individuals, the conscious Self whom we know or think we know, and behind him is a second individual that we may call the unconscious Self, or the sub-conscious or the imagination of whom we take no notice. But we are very wrong not to take notice of him, because it is he who guides us. If we can manage to guide this second individual CONSCIOUSLY, who up to the present has guided us, we shall then be able to guide ourselves.

"Here is a comparison that I will give you. Compare yourself to a person seated in a carriage, with a horse harnessed to it; but as if by mistake when harnessing it, we forgot to put on the reins. If you give the horse a touch with the whip and say: Gee up! the horse goes on; but where will he go? He goes anywhere he likes, to left, to right, forwards or backwards; and as he drags you behind him in the carriage, he takes you where it pleases him to go. Now if you can manage to put the reins on the horse, by this help you will be able to guide him to the place to which you wish to go, and as he draws you behind him, you will arrive at that place eventually. You will understand still better on seeing and trying some experiments.

EXPERIMENTS

"I will ask someone to establish consciously upon his mind this conflict between the will and the imagination: I wish to do such and such a thing, but I cannot do it! Now you, Mlle., will you try to experiment? Will you clasp your hands as tightly as you possibly can, until they begin to tremble; give me all your strength, I am greedy, I want it all! (The young girl stretches her arms in front of her and clasps her hands and locks them together until they tremble.) "There, now say to yourself: I will open my hands, but I CANNOT, I CANNOT! your hands lock tighter and tighter, always tighter!" (One sees the fingers of the girl lock themselves more tightly, her hands tremble, and her features contract with the effort she is making.) "Your hands are locked together as if they were always going to remain so, in spite of all your efforts, and the more you try to separate them, the more tightly they become locked! Now say to yourself: I CAN! (One sees that the girl's hands relax and drop apart.) "You see that it is sufficient to think a thing to make it become true, even if it is absurd! And truly, there is nothing more absurd than to think that you cannot open your hands and not be able to; just because you think: I CANNOT. (A patient.) "Yes, I understand, it is sufficient to say: I will, in order to become cured!"

M. Coué. "But you have not understood me at all! If you say to yourself; I will get well! your imagination, which is of a very contrary disposition, will most likely say: You "will" to be well, do you, well, my friend, you can go on expecting so! When you give the preference to the will, the imagination, which as I have said is very con-

trary, just thwarts you! Do not say therefore:
I WILL get well! But say: I am keeping on
getting better."

(The patient.) "All the specialists I have seen
up to the present have told me that I must exercise
my will!"

M. Coué. "Well, they have put their foot in
it, one and all!!!"

(Another patient, who is being treated for
insomnia.) "Yes, one of Bernheim's pupils also
told me to use the will; he tried to put me to
sleep for a year and a half, but without being able
to do so. Seeing that he was not able to obtain
any results, he said to me: You will never be
cured, you must put up with it and be contented
with your lot, and learn to bear your cross!"

M. Coué. "M. S. . . . suffered with insomnia
for 35 years, and for the last four nights he has
slept!"

(The patient.) "This morning I slept until six
o'clock; when I woke I thought it was eleven
o'clock at night and that I was going to have
another night of sleeplessness, but then I heard
the noises in the streets and found that it was
already morning!"

M. Coué. "Well let us return to our experi-

ments! Now, sir, you saw how Mlle. did the
experiment, will you stretch out your hands and
make the experiment for yourself. It is a very
good one, also the one with the stiff arm and
the clenched fist." (The experiment is made
upon the neurotic man; he does not understand
the idea of the experiment, and cannot keep his
hands closed.) "I am pleased that this hitch has
occurred, because many people believe that it de-
pends upon my will. I asked Monsieur to get into
a certain state of mind, but he has not known how
to do it; naturally the experiment cannot succeed!
Listen, you must try to make the experiment
thinking all the while: I CANNOT, and say
rapidly aloud: I CANNOT, CANNOT, CAN-
NOT! and while saying the word, try and unlock
your hands; and if you are really thinking: I
CANNOT, you will not be able to unclasp them.
There, that is good! As for me, I am always right
even when I seem to be wrong! For it is not what
I say that happens, it is what the person thinks!
What I wish to prove to you is that your thought
materializes. Only you must not try this experiment on yourself, as you might imagine it
has to be done, because you have to be in a certain state of mind such as I have asked of you

in order to succeed. When a person does not know how to think, or rather directs his thought badly, I teach him how to guide it by repeating CANNOT, CANNOT, very quickly so that he is unable to think: I CAN! You are not convinced, Sir, but you have taken notice of what I have said, and you laugh which is a good sign! Do not try to do this experiment alone, for generally you will not be in the right condition, the experiment will fail and you will lose confidence."

M. Coué then makes other experiments upon a child and a young man.

M. Coué (to a child). "Take this pen between your fingers and say to yourself: I would like to let it fall, but I CANNOT! (The child takes the pen and holds it, and tries to let it fall while thinking, I cannot. The more he thinks, I cannot, the tighter his fingers grasp it.) "Now think: I CAN! (the pen falls immediately to the ground)."

M. Coué (to another child). "Get up, my little man, you are going to try and give the little boy over there a blow of the fist on the head, saying to yourself: I would like to hit him, but I CANNOT! And you will not be able to do so; it will be as if a cushion were there which was stopping your fist from touching his head!"

M. Coué (to a young man). "Get up and say to yourself: My legs are stiff, I want to walk properly, but I CANNOT! As you say: CANNOT, try to walk; you cannot, you feel you will fall!" (The young man rises, stiffens his legs and tries to walk, but stumbles and is on the point of falling.) "Now say: I CAN walk!" (The young man loses his stiffness and begins to walk.) "Now say to yourself: I am glued to my chair, I would like to get up, but I CANNOT!" (The young man tries to rise while thinking: I cannot, but the greater the efforts he makes to rise, the more he appears fastened to his chair.) "Think now: I am no longer glued to my chair, I CAN rise!" (The young man rises easily from the chair.)

M. Coué. "You see that all ideas we put into the mind become a reality when they are within the limits of possibility, only you must always think in the right way and with continuity. If during a dozen seconds you think: I CANNOT, in the right way, and at the end of that time substitute the idea I CAN in the mind, then though your first thought was: I CANNOT, you will find that you can and the experiment will fail."

*

* *

THIRD PART

SUGGESTIONS: (a) GENERAL. (b)
SPECIAL FOR EACH AILMENT.

*

M. Coué addressing everyone:

"Now that you have really understood me, I am going to ask you to shut your eyes; so that you may not be disturbed by external objects; when the eyes are closed one is calmer, and one listens better!

"And say to yourselves that all the words I am going to say to you will fix, engrave and print themselves upon your mind, and that they will remain there always fixed, engraved and printed, and that this will happen without your will or knowledge, in fact, perfectly unconsciously on your part, and that you and your whole organism will obey them; because everything I am going to say is for your own good, and for the purpose of helping you, and therefore you will accept them all the more easily.

"I say to you that from now onwards all the physical functions of your body will improve with you, but particularly those of digestion, which are the most important. Therefore, three times each day regularly, in the morning, at mid-day and in the evening, you will be hungry and will eat with great pleasure, without, of course, eating

too much.   Above all you will be careful to masticate your food well.   (I speak to all, but more
especially to those persons suffering from the
liver, stomach or intestines), so be very careful to
masticate your food well, so that it is reduced to
a sort of soft paste before you swallow it.   In
these conditions digestion will be accomplished
easily, if not at once, then little by little it will
become so; and you will find that the sensations
of discomfort, heaviness nad pain in the stomach
that you have been in the habit of experiencing
will disappear gradually.

"And if any of you suffer from enteritis, you
will find that it will gradually diminish, that is
to say that the intestinal inflammation will disappear, and that the mucus or membrane which
accompanied it will also vanish.   If you have a
dilatation of the stomach, you will find that your
stomach will regain the elasticity and strength
which it has lost, that it will gradually resume its
normal size, and that it will execute more and
more easily those movements which pass the food
it contains into the intestines, and will thus facili-
tate intestinal digestion.

"Naturally as the digestion improves, assimilation will improve also (I say this for everyone,

but especially for those persons who are weakly)
your organism will profit by the food it receives
and will use it to make blood, muscles, strength,
energy, in fact life itself. You will find that day
by day you will become stronger and more vigorous, and that the feelings of weakness and weari-
ness which you have had will disappear, giving
place to a sense of strength and vigor; so that
should there be any anaemic condition in you,
your anaemia will leave you; your blood will become richer in quality and color and will take
on those qualities of the blood of a person who is
in good health. In these conditions anaemia is
bound to leave you, taking away with it all the
host of miseries that always follow in its train.

"I add for those persons whom it may concern,
that from now onwards the menstrual period will
take place normally. It will take place every 28
days, and will last 4 days neither more or less,
neither too much nor too little in quantity. You
will suffer no pain either before, during or after
its course, neither in the kidneys, pit of the
stomach, head nor anywhere else; and not only
will you not suffer pain, but you will not feel that
sort of nervous excitement which many women
experience at this time. In fact I tell you this

is essentially a natural function, and that it will take place normally and will not trouble you in any way at all.

"Naturally with the digestion and assimilation functioning properly, the evacuation of the bowels will take place very regularly. I must insist upon the point, for it is very important, because it is the *sine qua non* of good health. Therefore to-morrow, the day after tomorrow, and every day without exception, as soon as you get out of bed in the morning (or 20 minutes after breakfast, you may choose which you prefer) you will experience an imperative desire to evacuate the bowels; and you will always obtain a satisfactory result, without having to recourse to medicine or any artificial means whatever.

"I add that tonight, tomorrow night and every night in future, as soon as you wish to go to sleep, you will do so until that time in the morning at which you wish to awake; you will sleep calmly and soundly, without nightmare, so that when you awake you will feel very well, in fact gay, happy and quite rested. And you will always sleep in this way, in whatever place you may be, and in whatever circumstances you find yourself; and whatever the weather may be, whether it is

cold or hot, blows a gale or is calm, whether it
rains, snows or freezes, you will sleep a deep calm
sleep without nightmare; I do not say that your
sleep will be without dreams, but if you do dream
your dreams will be pleasant ones and will not
disturb you.

"Further, the digestion, assimilation, evacuation of the bowels, and sleep all being good, I say
that if you are in any way nervous, this nervousness will disappear and give place to a sensation
of peace, and you will find that you will become
gradually more and more master of yourself, both
from a physical as well as from a mental point
of view. All your symptoms will gradually disappear, or at least you will not experience them
so frequently, and the morbid feelings and fancies
that used to harass you formerly, will fade and
vanish.

"Finally and above all, and this is most essential for everyone, if up to the present you have
felt a certain distrust of yourself, this distrust
from now onwards, will gradually disappear, and
will give place to a feeling of confidence in yourself, YOU WILL HAVE CONFIDENCE IN
YOURSELF, you hear me, YOU WILL HAVE
CONFIDENCE IN YOURSELF. I repeat it,

and this confidence will enable you to do what you want to do well, even very well, whatever it may be, on condition, naturally, that it is reasonable (and it is reasonable to wish to obtain physical, mental and moral health). Therefore whenever you wish to do a thing that is reasonable, a thing which it is your duty to do, believe that as it is possible, the thing is easy. In consequence—such words as: Difficult . . . Impossible . . . I cannot . . . It is stronger than I . . . I cannot help it . . . I cannot prevent myself from . . . these words that we have constantly upon the lips, will disappear completely from your vocabulary; they are not English, understand me, they are NOT ENGLISH! What is English is: IT IS EASY . . . and I CAN! With these words you can accomplish absolute wonders. Believing that the thing which you wish to do is easy, it becomes so for you, although it may appear difficult to others. And you will do this thing quickly and well, with pleasure, without fatigue, without effort; while, on the other hand, had you considered it difficult or impossible, it would have become so for you, simply because you would have thought it so!"

*

* *

FOURTH PART

SPECIAL SUGGESTIONS FOR EACH AILMENT

Pain.—To those who have pain, in whatever part of the body it may be, in the foot, the leg, the knee, the back, the side, it does not matter where, I say to you that from this moment the cause of this pain, call it arthritis or by any other name, this cause will diminish and vanish, and the cause having disappeared, the effects which it caused will in their turn disappear also. And every time that I say to you that your pain is going, it is the same thing as a plane which takes a shaving of wood off the plank over which it is passed! And if this pain seems to come back sometimes, instead of thinking about it and bemoaning it as you used to do, say to yourself: I can send it away and without the least effort! But if you doubt it, you will not succeed, therefore be sure not to say: I will try and send it away! for to try expresses doubt. Therefore you will affirm to yourself that you can do this, and send the pain away (and this applies equally to mental and moral distress as well as physical). Therefore every time that you have a pain, physical or otherwise, you will go quietly to your room (it is better if you can do this, but you can do it also in the middle of the road if necessary), but if you go to your room, sit down and shut your eyes, pass your hand lightly across your forehead if it is mental distress, or upon the part that hurts if it is pain in any part of the body, and repeat the words: It is going, it is going, etc. Very rapidly, even at the risk of gabbling, it is of no importance. The essential idea is to say: it is going, it is going, so quickly, that it is impossible for a thought of contrary nature to force itself between the words. We thus actually think it is going, and as all ideas that we fix upon the mind become a reality for us, the pain, physical or mental vanishes. And should the pain return, repeat the process 10, 20, 50, 100, 200 times if necessary, for it is better to pass the entire day saying: It is going! than to suffer pain and complain about it. Be more patient than your pain, drive it back to its last entrenchments! And you will find that the more you use this process, the less you will have to, that is to say, that if today you use it 50 times, tomorrow you will only use it 48, and the next day 46 and so on . . . so that at the end of a relatively short space of time, you will have no need to use it at all.

Lungs: And for those persons who have any

trouble with the lungs, I tell you that your organism will become ever stronger and more vigorous, thanks to your improved powers of assimilations, and that it will find within itself those elements which are necessary to repair any lesions which may exist in the lungs, bronchial tubes and chest. In proportion as these lesions heel, you will find that the symptons from which you have suffered will diminish, and will end by disappearing completely. If you have expectorations, you will find that they will gradually diminish in quantity and will become more and more easy; if you suffer from a feeling of oppression, this will become more and more rare; if you cough, your fits of coughing will become less and less violent, less frequent, and will finally disappear completely and absolutely.

Eyes: To those persons who suffer from their eyes, I say that any lesions you may have in the eyes will heal little by little, and will finally disappear, so that the eyes will gradually become better and better, that is to say, that every day you will see further, more clearly and more sharply.

Myopia: And for you, Mlle., who suffer from myopia, your crystalline lens which is too elongated, and which reflects the image in front of the retina, will flatten little by little; the image will gradually be produced further and further away, and at the end of a certain time the lens will have its normal thickness, and the sight will be normal.

Incontinence in Children: As for you, my child, the accident that happens to you at night, will not happen again. It has not occurred for a fortnight and it will not occur again. From now onwards every time that you wish to urinate, you will wake up, always, ALWAYS; when you awake you will accomplish this duty at once, and directly you get back into bed, as soon as your head touches the pillow, you will fall asleep and sleep soundly until the morning, or until another desire to get up awakens you, and you will get up, but will sleep again directly. Now you can consider yourself cured, but go on with your suggestion, say always: Everyday and in every way I am getting better and better. What you think will produce itself, and you will benefit from it all your life.

Lameness in a Child: As for you, my little one, whose right leg is not so strong as the other, your organism will become stronger and stronger and will find within itself all those elements which are necessary to cause the formation of new muscular cells, which, adding themselves to those cells, which are already there, will increase the size of those muscles and will make them stronger; and little by little your leg will become fatter. Every day you will notice that the slight limp you have will become less and less, and will end by disappearing completely.

Nervous Fits: And for you who have nervous fits, you must not have any more and you will not have them; and if in spite of all, a fit seems to be coming on, you will always know it beforehand, ALWAYS, you hear what I say; and it will produce certain symptoms which will warn you, and you will hear a voice, MINE, which will say to you as quickly as lightning: You will have not this fit, it is going, it has gone! And the fit will have disappeared before it even had the time to make its appearance.

Children's Studies: And for all you children, I say that from now onwards you will be good children, obedient, attentive to your parents, grand-parents, uncles and masters, in fact towards everyone who has a right to your respect and your obedience. When they tell you to do something or make a remark, I know that you

will take notice of it.   Generally when anyone
tells children to do something or make a remark,
they are apt to think that it is done or said to
annoy them, to "bore" them, as you say!   But
now you know that when anyone reproaches or
reprimands you, it is not done to annoy you, but
that it is done for your own good.   And far from
having a grudge against the person who made
the remark to you, you will be grateful to him
for having made it.   And further, I say, that you
will like work, YOU WILL LIKE YOUR
WORK, and as the work which you have to do
at present consists entirely of your studies, you
will like to study all those things which you have
to learn, and especially those that you do not care
for at present.   Generally children imagine that
they do not like certain lessons and they say: Oh!
I loathe arithematic, I hate history!   They only
hate it because they imagine they do; but if you
thought, on the contrary, that you would like a
certain lesson, you will like it!   And the proof of
this is that in the future, you will notice that you
will learn everything very easily, and that you will
like all your lessons; so that from now onwards
when you are in school and the master is explain-
ing a lesson, you will keep your attention fixed

on everything he says, without taking any notice of the stupid things that your companions may be doing or saying, and without doing them yourself. And as you are clever, you hear me, YOU ARE CLEVER, you will understand what you learn, and you will place everything in the storehouse of your memory, from whence you will draw them when you have need of them. When you work alone, in school or at home, you will keep your whole attention fixed exclusively upon the duty which you have to perform, or on the lesson which you have to learn, and thus your work will always be irreproachable.

Liver: And for those persons who have anything the matter with the liver, I say that from this moment your organism and your unconscious Self will do all that is necessary in order to heal any lesions that may exist; and if there is simply some abnormality, that this abnormality will disappear. In both cases your organism will function normally; it will secrete the necessary amount of bile of right quality, and it will flow naturally into the intestines where it aids intestinal digestion. And particularly for those who suffer from hepatic colic, I say that from now onwards your liver will secrete alkaline bile instead of acid bile as it used to do; this acid bile, as I told you before, leaves a deposit in the bile duct which accumulates and forms gallstones; if you have at the present moment a collection of these gallstones; it is probable that they will not dissolve, and that every time they pass into the bile duct, they will give you colic, but as soon as you have got rid of them all, they will not form again.

Heart: And for those persons who have anything the matter with the heart, I say that from this moment your organism and your unconscious Self will do what is necessary to cause the lesion which you may have to disappear; your heart will function normally, the circulation will improve, and the unpleasant palpitations will become gradually more, and more rare, and will finally disappear completely.

Child's Heart: For you, my child, I say that the sore place you have in your heart will go away; (to the child's mother). It is very probable that the lesion will remain in the heart, but the organism will do what is necessary to establish a sort of compensation, so that although the child will not be cured, she will no longer suffer, and will be able to do everything that other people do. It is the same as a case I had of a boy whom

I treated in 1912. He was not cured, because he was invalided twice during the war on account of his heart, but he can ride a bicycle, play football, and goes for excursions. And the proof that he suffers no longer is that he was married three months ago!

Lesions of the Brain. Paralysis: As for you, Mlle. I say that those lesions which have occurred in your brain (caused by encephilitis) ; and which are getting better, will continue to do so; in proportion as they disappear you will find that the symptoms which they produce will also vanish; that fatigue and lassitude which makes you seem dull, will gradually diminish and disappear; the feeling of emptiness which you experience will give place to one of strength and vigor; YOU WILL WANT TO WORK, you must work, even if it is only to dig a hole in the garden and then another one to fill up the first. IT IS ABSOLUTELY NECESSARY THAT YOU SHOULD FEEL THE DESIRE TO WORK! Your mother tells you to work, and I am speaking through her, it is I, I, who speak to you, and (in an imperative tone of voice) if you were with me, I should insist that you should.

The Nose: And for you, Sir, who are suffering from the nose, I say that your organism and your unconscious Self will do all that is necessary in order that this slight lesion, or rather the irration that you feel in the nose will disappear; you will find that your chronic bronchitis will grow less and in time will disappear; as for your asthma there is no need to speak of that for it is cured, QUITE CURED!

Pains in the Legs: For you, I say that you will find the pains which you have in the legs will disappear, and they will not leave you for a short time only, but entirely. Do not fear their return, above all; say to yourself. They will not come back! And you will find that the stiffness which you feel will disappear, and that the pains you have in the stomach will also diminish; if you have any internal trouble your unconscious Self will do all that is necessary to make it disappear.

Kidneys, Bladder: For those persons who may have lesions in the kidneys or bladder, I say that these lesions will be cured little by little, and after some time they will be completely cured and will disappear; you will no longer suffer any sort of pain, more or less violent as you have been accustomed to, in either the kidneys or bladder;

your urine will become normal and will no longer contain a deposit.

Gravel: For those who suffer from gravel, I say the nourishment of your body will continue to improve and will become more normal and regular; the kidneys will no longer form an excess of uric acid, and you will help them by drinking a large amount of liquid, the more you take, the less likely will be the formation of uric acid crystals, and in consequence you will suffer less pain.

Depression: And for those who suffer from depression, I say that every day you are becoming better and better; this depression will grow less and less, and will give place to a sensation of physical and mental strength such as you never hoped to possess; and you will become completely master of yourself both physically and mentally. The time will come when you will be able to work all day long without feeling tired, but you must take care not to make any efforts, and also to conserve your strength, instead of wasting it as you have been doing.

Tumor on the Tongue: And for you, Sir, who had a growth on the tongue which necessitated a surgical operation, I say to you that your organ-

ism will do all that is necessary in order to cause
these parasitical cells to disappear; they will be
replaced by perfectly healthy cells, which will
repair the damage done by the unhealthy cells.

Abscess: And to any persons who may have
an abscess, I say that your organism will do all
that is necessary in order to make them gradually
disappear; the inflammation will subside, the
quantity of pus will diminish each day, the scar
will form, and a complete cure will follow.

Tremblings: And for those persons whom it
concerns, I say that whatever may be the nature
of the lesions that you may have in the brain or
the nervous system, and which have caused the
symptoms which you have had . . . stiffness and
trembling, and the difficulty you have of keeping
upright, the pains in the back and the slight
paralysis you have of the right side . . . I tell you
that these lesions will heal gradually day by day,
and will continue to do so, and the cause of the
trouble will disappear, so that the effects which
it has produced will also disappear in the same
proportion. You will find that the stiffness will
diminish and that you will be able to hold yourself erect more and more easily; the trembling
which you feel in the hand and arm will lesson,

you will feel yourself becoming stronger and stronger and more and more sure of yourself; when you walk, walk slowly with rather long steps, taking care to separate the legs; when you advance the left leg, place it before the right one, and when you advance the right leg, place it before the left one; in this way you will keep your balance.

Varicose Veins: To those persons who have varicose veins, I say that your organism and your unconscious Self will do all that is necessary in order to establish a sort of compensation; the tissue of your veins will resume their normal strength and consistency; but it is not sufficient that the veins be cured, the varicose ulcer must also be cured. I say that your organism will do all that is necessary to build up a series of healthy bells within the wound, so that it will disappear, the edges of the wound will gradually draw together, a scar will form, and the cure will be complete.

Phlebitis: I say to those persons suffering from phlebitis, that your organism and your unconscious Self will do all that is necessary in order to establish a sort of compensation; in phlebitis the larger vein is blocked by a clot of blood, and naturally the blood does not flow in as quickly as it flows out; this causes a swelling; therefore your unconscious Self will do all that is necessary to establish compensation, that is, a vein beside the affected one will enlarge so as to permit a free flow of the blood.

Hernia: For you who suffer from hernia, I say that from now onwards your organism and your unconscious Self will do all that is necessary in order to gradually form a scar in the peritoneal tissue which was ruptured; your intestine used to pass through this passage and produce the hernia; from now onwards your unconscious Self will gradually cause the ruptured tissue to heal up from either end (of the kind of button-hole which exists), so that it will become smaller and smaller, and the hernia will be reduced in size, when the closing of the hole is complete, the hernia will have disappeared.

Growths: For those persons who have an excrescene of growth, of whatever nature they may be, whether is be of a fibrous nature or a gland ... I say that your organism and your unconscious Self will do all that is necessary in order to cause the disappearance of these parasitical cells; in proportion as their destruction is carried out, the growth will lose a proportional amount of its size and hardness, and when reabsorbtion is complete, the growth will have disappeared.

Loss of Memory: To those persons who complain of loss of memory, I say that you have lost your memory simply because you have thought you have done so! Loss of memory only occurs because one thinks it is lost! You have only to think that your memory will return and it will!

Vices, (Drink) Etc.: And for those who feel strongly attracted by certain things, I say this attraction will be replaced by an equally strong repulsion, and the trouble from which you suffered will end.

Doubts: For those who suffer from doubts, I say that the incretitude and doubts from which you have suffered will give place to a feeling of certitude and you will find that which you seek.

Sad Thoughts and Ideas: For those persons who have sad thoughts and ideas, I say that from now onwards these thoughts will become more and more rare; they will become less tenacious and will cease to cling to you; and every time that they may return, you will employ the process: It is going, it is going! Put them outside the door of your mind with all the honors due to them! But I want you to realize that it is not I who can cure you, it is you who must do so, and upon yourself only depends your cure. And this is of great importance for you, for if I were a healer (and I have explained to you that I am not), once you were no longer here, or I was no longer with you, I could no longer help you; if however, on the contrary, you realize that you possess within yourself the power of healing yourself, you have only to use it every time that it is necessary. Further, if you have a tendency to melancholy, this tendency will decrease and give place to one of gaiety; if you feel yourself haunted, followed or pursued by unhealthy ideas, fears, aversions or by any morbid ideas that are capable of harming you, I say that these ideas will pass from your mind, will become as a distant cloud, and will finally disappear completely. And if instead of fearing these thoughts you look them squarely in the face and laugh at them, you will have them no more! And above all, do not say as one is so often in the havit of saying: I am too old . . . I shall never get over it . . . It has lasted too long . . . I shall always suffer in this way . . . and other things of the same nature, it is ABSURD! You must say to yourself that which is true: (and which will become all the more quickly and completely true the more you think of it), . . . I am on the road to recovery . . . I am getting better! Every day will add a fresh stone to the edifice of your health, and in a short time you will be completely cured; this is the state of mind in which you must remain and which will enable you to make rapid progress toward the way to health and make it quickly and completely.

I am going to count three, and when I say "three", you will come out of the state in which you are, you will come out of it very quietly, you will be perfectly wideawake, not dazed at all, nor tired, but will feel full of life and health; and you will always feel thus, healthy and well both physically and mentally. I count three, ONE . . . TWO . . . THREE.

*

* *

FIFTH PART

ADVICE TO PATIENTS.

"Well now, I have given you some very good advice! And in order to make this advice a reality I say, for *AS LONG AS YOU LIVE!* (I am exacting, I do not ask it for one day, or a month, or a year, but for ALL your life), every morning before rising and every night when you are in bed, you will shut your eyes and you will repeat 20 times with the lips, loud enough to hear yourself (and in order to save yourself from counting, make a sort of rosary with a piece of string in which you have tied 20 knots, so that you count automatically), the following little sentence: *EVERY DAY AND IN EVERY WAY I AM GETTING BETTER AND BETTER!* And when you say this sentence do not think of anything in particular, the words "in every way" apply to everything. The essential thing is that you say these words very simply, as a child would, in a very monotonous tone of voice, and above all, ABOVE ALL, without *EFFORT,* that is the essential condition, say these words as one says a litany in church, it is the best example I can give you, thus: Every day, etc. . . . . By its repetition you will come to impress upon your mind the idea that *EVERY DAY AND IN EVERY WAY I AM GETTING BETTER AND BETTER.* You have seen by the explanations which I have given you and by the experiments which you have made, that every idea which we put into the mind becomes a reality, as long as it is within the limits of possibility; therefore if you impress upon your mind the idea that you will be cured, a cure will follow as a matter of course, and the contrary will be produced if you impress upon the mind the idea that you are ill.

"Autosuggestion is a double-edged weapon; well used it works wonders, badly used it brings nothing but disaster. Up to the present you have wielded this weapon unconsciously, and made bad suggestions to yourselves, but that which I have taught you will prevent from ever again making bad autosuggestions, and if you should do so, you can only beat yourself upon the breast, and say: It is my own fault; entirely my own fault!

And do not say when you are well: Oh! I am all right now, it is useless to go with my suggestion! Tell yourself on the contrary, that it is easier to prevent an evil than it is to cure it. How long does it take to break a leg? There is a piece of orange peel upon the pavement, you step on it, slip; fall and break a leg; how long does that take? One second, no longer! But how long will it take to repair the damage, even with suggestion? Weeks!!! If you had not broken your leg, you would not have had the trouble of healing it; therefore every time that you say your suggestion, tell yourself that you brush a piece of orange peel out of your way, and so in this manner you prevent yourself breaking a limb, either physically or mentally!

If you use your suggestions *CONSCIEN-TIOUSLY* you will perform wonders. For the result, I do as Mr. Pontius Pilate of illustrious memory did, I wash my hands of you; *IT DE-PENDS ENTIRELY UPON YOURSELF!*

*
* *

SIXTH PART

AD VERBATIM REPORT OF LECTURE DELIVERED BY EMILE COUÉ IN VARIOUS PARTS OF THE UNITED STATES ON HIS VISIT HERE IN JANUARY-FEBRUARY, 1923.

*

Ladies and gentlemen, first of all I must pray you to excuse me not to speak English so well as I would desire to do, but you know I have been born a Frenchman. I never lived in England nor in America, and it is pretty difficult, for such a man to speak English as well as you do, but I hope you will be able to understand me.

I must say to you, first, that I don't know how to thank you for the reception you make me. I am quite confused, but I thank you from my heart. The best I think I can do is to give you in a few words the principles of the method I have instituted in Nancy, owing to which results have been obtained which others have not been able to obtain.

When people come and see me I tell them first, most of them in coming to me think they will find an extraordinary man. You see, he is not extraordinary. They think they will find a man endowed with an extraordinary power, a sort of magic power, owing to which he is able to cure people making as I do now (motioning with the hands). I am not the man you think I am, not

at all.   I am not a healer, as many people call me;
I am not a magic maker, not in the least.

I am only a man, a very simple man, as you see;
a good man, if you like, but only a man.   My part
is not to heal people, but to teach them what they
can do to heal themselves, or at least to improve
themselves, and to show them that they will get
this result by using an instrument which we use
all our lives long without knowing it—I will say
autosuggestion.

Autosuggestion is an instrument which we
possess at our birth, and from that time, from the
first day of our birth, we use this instrument during the night, during the day.   All our dreams
are the result of autosuggestion.   All that we do,
all that we say, is also the result of autosuggestion, unconscious autosuggestion.

You think perhaps that I exaggerate.   I do not
exaggerate.   We use this instrument at the first
day of our birth.   Here is an example I usually
give.   A young baby, two days old, lies in its
cradle.   All at once it cries.

One of the parents takes it from its cradle.
The baby ceases crying.   The parent puts it again
into its cradle, and immediately it cries again.

The parent takes it a second time from its cradle. The baby ceases crying, and so on.

The baby is trying to make suggestion to his parents, and very often he succeeds. Unfortunately for the parents, if the parents make themselves the autosuggestion that it is necessary for them to take the baby from its cradle every time it cries, as a consequence it is necessary to spend one year or more to 'have the baby in the arms instead of in the bed, where it would be much better, and the baby says to himself, "Every time I shall desire to be taken from my cradle, I shall cry," and he cries. Isn't that true?

If on the contrary the parents let the baby cry a minute, a quarter of an hour, half an hour, one hour, the baby thinks it is not necessary to cry, it is no use, and he doesn't do it again.

As I told you before, this instrument, autosuggestion, we use it all our lifetime, but we use it unconsciously. Autosuggestion is a very beneficial instrument when it is used well, properly. It produces very often wonderful effects. It produces what is called miracles. When it is used wrongly, badly, it can produce disasters.

My part is to show people that they are this

instrument in themselves, and to teach them how to use it consciously. When you use a dangerous instrument consciously, the instrument ceases to be dangerous. The danger resides in the ignorance of the danger. When the danger is known, that is not so. It is my part to show you how it can be done, that it is a very, very simple thing. It is so simple that it is difficult to think that such a simple thing produces such wonderful effects.

After having spoken so, before giving you counsel, because I give counsels without making suggestions, I don't make any suggestions. I don't use hypnotism—I can say that because I began by studying hypnotism and practising it during a few years, and little by little I have ceased. I have abandoned this way, and I have used the method which I will expose to you.

Before giving you counsel, after which I will make upon you some experiments which will show you the two principles upon which I have built my theory, I will explain to you my method of conscious autosuggestion.

Do you hear me well?

(A Voice). Talk a little louder.

M. Coué. Thank you, I will do it. This experiment will show you the two things upon which I have built my theory of conscious autosuggestion. The first one is this:

Every idea we have in our mind becomes a reality, in the domain of possibility. If a thing is realizable, it takes place; we must not put such ideas into our mind, unless we feel it is possible for them to take place.

For instance, if you have a leg cut off, and you imagine the leg will grow again, it is positive it will not grow again, because till now we are not able to produce such miracles; but if we have sad ideas, if we have organs which do not work well, if we have pain in a part of our body and we imagine that the sad ideas will be replaced by pink ideas, that our organs will, little by little, function better; that the pain we have, in whatever part of the body, will disappear, it takes place, because it is possible.

The idea of sleep creates sleep; the idea of sleeplessness creates sleeplessness. What is a person who sleeps well? It is a person who knows that when one is in the bed it is for sleep, and he sleeps. What is a person who does not sleep during the night? It is a person who knows that when one is in the bed it is not for to sleep. The person knows when he goes to bed that he will not sleep better this night than the preceding night.

The idea of nervous crises creates nervous crises. The idea of a bad headache on the day when one is invited to dinner at madame so-and-so's, creates a bad headache precisely on the day. If a person is invited on Monday, it is on Monday that he gets his bad headache. If it is on Thursday, it is on Thursday that he gets his bad headache.

It is sufficient to think, "I am blind," "I am deaf," "I am paralyzed," to be deaf, blind or paralyzed. I will not say that all the people who are deaf, blind or paralyzed are so because they think they are, but there are many who are so only because they think they are. I can show it to you because I have seen such people, and it is with these people that the so-called miracles take place.

My merit, if I have a merit, is not a great one. I have succeeded to cure a man or a person who was not ill. It happens very often, very often.

I will give you an example. Last year, at the beginning of the year, a young lady came in to see me at Nancy. She was 23 years old. Since the age of 3 years she could not see anything with her left eye, absolutely nothing.

Immediately after the meeting she saw, as you see, with the left eye.   People who were present thought it was a miracle.   It was no miracle, and I will explain to you.   It is very easy.

When the young lady was a child, 2 years old, she got a pain, she got an illness in her left eye, and this illness required about a year to be cured. During that time she was obliged to have a bandage on her left eye, and during that time also the eye took the habit of not to see, and when the bandage was taken off the eye preserved the habit of not to see, and this lasted 20 years.   It would last till now if she had not come to me.   I persuaded her that she could see, and as it was possible, she saw.   She, understand, she was very easy to understand.

I have seen the same case, or nearly the same case, with a paralytic woman.   It was in Paris. They brought her to me, on the first floor.   She could not make the least movement with her right side.   Immediately after the meeting she stood up, walked and moved her bad arm as well as the other one.

People thought it was a miracle.   It was no

miracle, and it is easy to explain. I think that at the beginning she got a true paralysis, she got a stroke. There was a clot there.

At this moment the paralysis was true, but little by little, as it happens very often, the clot disappeared, diminished, and, of course, the true paralysis diminished also in the same proportion, but the woman always thought, "I am paralyzed," and she continued to be paralyzed.

Later on the clot disappeared completely. At that moment the true paralysis disappeared also, but she continued to have in her mind the idea, "I am paralyzed," and she remained paralyzed. I persuaded her she could make the movements she desired to make, and she made them.

What is the conclusion we may draw from this first statement? Every idea we have in our minds becomes a reality, in the domain of possibility. Being ill, we put in our minds the idea of healing. Healing takes place if healing is possible; if healing is not possible, it does not take place, but in such a case we get the greatest improvement it is possible to obtain.

I will not say that the use of conscious autosuggestion must prevent people to take the medicines they are accustomed to take, or to follow the orders of their doctors. Autosuggestion and medicine must not be considered as enemies.

On the contrary, they must be considered as good friends, which must help each other, and I can tell you one of my greatest desires is to introduce in the schools of medicine the study of autosuggestion, for the benefit of the doctors and therefore for the great benefit of their patients.

It is not will-power which is the first quality of man, but imagination. I repeat it, because it is a point in which my method differs from all other methods, and owing to which I can obtain results where the other methods have failed. It is not will power which is the first quality of man, but imagination.

Every time there is a conflict between will power and imagination, it is always imagination which has the best of it, always, without any exception, and in such cases when we say, "I want to do such and such a thing, but I can't do it," not only we don't do what we are desiring to do, but we do exactly the contrary of what we are desiring to do, and the greater the will power is, the more we do the contrary of what we are desiring to do. I will show you that I am right

in giving you some examples which I have chosen
from my life.

I take for the first example, sleeplessness.
Some of you shall say that I am right. If a
person who does not sleep during the night, does
not want to sleep, does not make any effort to
sleep, but lies very quiet in his bed, without
moving, he will sleep; if on the contrary, the
person who wants to sleep makes an effort to
sleep, what happens? When a person tries to
sleep, the more he is excited, and this person does
not do exactly what he wants to do. This person
tries to find sleep, and he finds—wakefulness—
which is the contrary of sleep. This example is
known by every one of you.

So also the forgetting of a name. If it hasn't
happened to you, it may still happen. Every time
you want to find the name of Mrs.—what's her
name, you know—the less you can find it. Generally, after a minute it comes back, but it is
necessary to analyze this phenomenon, which contains two phenomena.

You come home and say to your wife or
husband, or sister or brother, or your mother,
"Well, I just met Mrs."—you hesitate. This

hesitation creates in your mind the idea, "I have forgotten."

As every idea we have in our mind becomes a reality, and as you have this idea in your mind, you cannot find the name. You may try, but you cannot. You may run, but the name will run more quickly than you, and you shall not be able to catch it. That has happened to every one of you.

Generally, after a few minutes it comes when one ceases trying to find the name, and you say it will soon come back. The idea, "I have forgotten," disappeared, after having been replaced by the idea, "It will come back," which in its turn comes true, and while conversing you interrupt yourself to say, "Oh, it is Mrs. So-and-so." That is an example that is well known.

Take uncontrollable laughter. Under certain circumstances the more we try not to laugh, the more we laugh. The more the motorcyclist tries to avoid an obstacle on the track, the straighter it runs into him.

It has happened to many of you, I am sure. The more the stammerer tries not to stammer, the more he stammers, and so on, which puts me in mind of the person in such circumstances who says, "I want to sleep, but I cannot," or the one who says, "I want to find the name of Mrs. So-and-so, but I cannot," "I want to prevent me from stammering, but I cannot." It is always, "I cannot."

The imagination is always the best in its conflict with will power. It is imagination that is the first quality of man, and not the second one. You must know that we have in ourselves two beings. The first one is the conscious, voluntary being which we know, and the second one, behind the first being, is another one, the subconscious or imaginative being, or imagination, as you call it.

We don't pay attention to this being, and we are perfectly wrong, because it is this second being which runs us entirely.

We all have organs in this part of our body, we have a heart, we have a stomach, we have kidneys, we have a liver, and so on.

No one of us has any power upon those organs by his own will power, no one. However, those organs work; they work even during the night, when the conscious being is asleep. They work under the influence of the first. The first is the subsconscious or unconscious mind. Not only does this unconscious being run, preside over the functions of these organs, but it presides also over all the functions of our physical body, and our moral body, if I can use this expression.

If it is the second being which runs us, and we learn how to run it, through it we learn how to run ourselves. Do you understand? I repeat, because it is the principal thing. It is our unconscious being which runs us. We learn how to run it. Through it we learn to run ourselves.

It is a sort of little trick. When one learns the trick he is able to become master of himself. I suppose you have understood. You will understand better in seeing some experiments which I generally make—not generally, I always make—with people, to let them see, to let them feel that what I say is the truth.

I will show the experiment on myself, and afterwards I shall make it with some persons who will come to me. I will establish consciously a conflict between my imagination and my will power. I will press my hands together as tight as I can, and put into my mind the idea, "I cannot open it." Now, that I have put this idea into my mind, the idea that I cannot open my hands, the more I try to open them the tighter I press.

And now I am ill. It is a true illness that I have. It is called contraction, and you have seen in your life, every one of you, people who are ill in the same manner. You have seen people who could not open their hands, for instance, or close them, or you have seen people who walk with a leg stiff, as if it were wood. Out of a hundred, 80 I think cannot do the movements they are desiring to do because they think they cannot, and they remains all their life long in this state, if they preserve in their minds the idea, "I cannot."

To cure myself when I am ill, I must replace in my mind the idea "I cannot" by the idea "I can," and immediately I will feel that I am able to.

(At this point M. Coué gave a demonstration, using the above formula.)

You see, you think I am doing it on purpose. I am doing it on purpose, to show you what it is, but the experiment is quite true, and I will make this experiment with one or two or three persons here, if you will be so kind.

Presiding Officer: Ladies and gentlemen,

a number of times when M. Coué has asked
for these experiments, some people have thought
they were proposed as having some mysterious
power, and some people who were more or less
influenced have come forward, but I trust you
will understand that this is simply a demonstration of the power of the imagination over the
will, and if perhaps two or three from this side
of the table come forward who will be interested
to demonstrate, and two or three from this side,
just in order that he may show you what he
means by this power of the imagination over the
will.

(Several of those seated at the speaker's table
offered themselves for the demonstration.)

M. Coué: In this experiment it is not what
I shall say which will take place, but what the
person will think.   If they think well, as I shall
pray them to do, it will take place.   If they think
the contrary, the contrary will take place.   I don't
try to oblige people to make these experiments.
It is no hypnotism, it is no suggestion on my part,
it is only autosuggestion on the part of the person,
hence you will laugh at me, but it doesn't matter.
In every case I am right.

What is my meaning?   I will show you that

when we have an idea in our minds, this idea becomes very eloquent. I tell the person to close his hands and to think, "I cannot open them." If I see that the person presses his hands tighter and tighter and thinks, "I cannot," I am right, he cannot open his hands.

If, on the contrary, after I have said to the person to think, "I cannot," he opens his hands, he has thought "I can." Am I not right? You understand. It is difficult to say the contrary. I ask every person if he understands me, because if the person does not understand, of course it does not take place.

(Addressing a lady at the speaker's table:) Put your arms out straight and stiff, please. Press your hands together as tight as you can. Give me your strength. A little more, a little more, a little more, a little more. Give me all your strength. Your hands must tremble. Say to yourself, "I want to open my hands, but I cannot," and press tighter and tighter. Think now "I can."

Now will you grasp your fist as tight as you can. To succeed one must give all one's strength. Look at it now and think, "I want to open my hand, but I cannot, I cannot, I cannot," and press tighter and tighter. Think now "I can." I pray the person to think, but if the person would think the contrary, the contrary would take place. I don't know whether you understand or not.

Now will you put your hands together, please, always as tight as you can. Look at them now and think, "I want to separate my hands, but I cannot separate them," then when you try to separate them, the tighter they press. Think now "I can."

You are a good subject. Very often in public it is not the same. When people come to me at Nancy they come with confidence. Generally the experiment does not fall. In your country it is not the same. Your people do not believe, there is a certain diffidence, and often—I don't say often—but yesterday every experiment has succeeded, and I hope it will be the same today. It is to be understood that people are not accustomed to be in public.

Now will you suspend this key ring with your two fingers, and press as tight as you can and say, "I can't drop it," and you cannot, you press tighter and tighter. Think now "I can." You can easily do it.

Will you put your hand on the table, and press

as much as you can and say, "Now I can no longer lift my hand, I cannot, I cannot," and the more you try the less you can, you press tighter and tighter. Think now "I can." Thank you.

(The experiments were repeated with a number of others in the audience.)

Generally when a person intends to succeed in his field he takes a precaution to cultivate his field, because he knows well that if he does not take this precaution the seed will not grow. I do the same with people. When people come to me I think of them as uncultivated fields. I plow them by giving the explanation I have given you, by making the demonstrations I have shown you, and when they are cultivated I can sow my seed, and the seed will grow, I sow my seed by making a little discourse.

In English I tell them that the functions of the body will go rightly, they will have a good appetite, digestion will take place properly, assimilation will be good, they will sleep well every night.

I will not make you a discourse, it will be too long. When I have given this counsel I tell people I will count three, and when I say three you open your eyes, and you feel quite well. I tell them to close their eyes to hear what I say to them. They open their eyes generally on people, smiling, and after a while you see I have given you good counsel, I have done my part; now you must do yours, and it is what you must do, if you will profit by my counsels.

As long as you live, every morning, before getting up, every night, as soon as you are lying in bed, shut your eyes, and repeat 20 times, with your lips, loud enough to hear your own words, without trying to think of what you are saying— if you think of it, it is well; if you don't think of it, it is well—counting it on a little string, providing yourself with a little string of knots, "Day by day, in every way, I am getting better and better."

In this little phrase there are three important words, "In every way," which impute all the suggestion. Thus it is quite useless to make particular suggestions, as they are all included in three words "in every way," but you must pay attention to make the suggestion, the autosuggestion, very simply.

Try it like this, in a monotonous manner, without any effort, as they recite the litanies in the church, "Day by day, in every way, I am getting better and better," and so on, till 20.

By repetition you succeed to put into your mind, unconscious mind, mechanically through the ear, the phrase, "Day by day, in every way, I am getting better and better."

You have seen by the explanations I have given you and the experiments I have made with you, that when we have an idea in our mind this idea becomes a reality. Thus if you think, "Every day, in every way, I am getting better and better," day by day, in every way, you are getting better and better.

You see, it is very simple, it is very easy, as I repeat, too simple to be well understood the first time.

Now, finally, to show you the results such a custom can do, I will ask you the permission to read before you one or two letters, to show you what that method can do.

Will you allow me?

"Dear M. Coué—In 1920 I met with an accident, causing concussion and paralysis. I consulted a specialist, who did nothing of any value, but an open minded and advanced medical man took my case in hand and sent me for a rest cure in the country. In six months I could only walk a hundred yards in one hour, and had not mental balance. I took up your treatment of autosuggestion, after reading reports of your wonderful work. In a short time only, following what I have read, I am now wonderfully well, and walked nine miles."

Another one which has been written to a lady, and given to me: "Am just steadily getting better and better"—there is the formula—"in fact, many people have been converted to believe in autosuggestion, just by seeing me and my improved health. People all say they hardly know me, I look so different, so much better. I don't think I ever remember feeling so well."

The last one: "Dear M. Coué: I am sure it will interest you to know that I am very much better since I was at Nancy, and attended your lectures in July. You will perhaps remember me by the fact that I had been actually sick at least once a day for 10 years. The sickness stopped after I had been a week at Nancy and has not come back."

You see, I can assure you that if you will make every morning and every night the autosuggestion which I have given you the counsel to do, you will get better in every way, and for the business it gives a strong, an enormous strength, because you get confidence in yourself, and when you have confidence in yourself you will succeed.   I wish to profit you by my counsels, and I thank you for the attention you have given me.